Yama Niyama

Yogic Ethics for a Balanced Mind

Yama Niyama

Avt. Ananda Tapasiddha Ac.

Other books by the same author:

'Ink of the Heart: Mystical Songs of Prabhat Rainjain Sarkar'

'Intangible Things Set Free' (Poetry)

To all those who continue to believe that it is worthwhile to keep making the effort to become better people, and that this is an essential part of being human.

CONTENTS

INTRODUCTION

To understand an idea, it is always necessary to grasp not only its appearance but also its inner spirit. Upon this a proper conceptualization of the given topic can be gained, and for this one must know the context in which it sits. To realize the purpose and meaning of the guidelines of behaviour which Yama-Niyama are, the same must be applied. In fact, one of the points of the Niyamas, 'Svádhyáya', suggests exactly this: that one must read with proper perception, grasping not only what is literally being said, but what is implied, the essence of the words. This small book is an attempt to explain the teachings of Yama-Niyama in such a way, prompting a process of self-reflection which can serve towards the deepening of our ethical, emotional and spiritual lives both individually and collectively.

Yama-Niyama are basically a set of ten 'ethical guidelines', divided equally into two parts: the 'Yamas' and the 'Niyamas.' The five points of the Yamas are designed to establish a balanced relationship between the inner and outer worlds, the subjective and objective, and are distinguished from the Niyamas in that they cannot be implemented without an external object to be acted upon. The Niyamas are internal attitudes which can be cultivated without the need of a second entity.[1] Originating in the Indian subcontinent, the Yamas and Niyamas are well known for being included in the yoga sutras of Patainjali, but like many other ideas in that book by no means originated there. Similar and also other somewhat different different versions can be found recorded and interpreted in numerous ancient texts and were surely taught orally, as was the system of basically all Indian spiritual traditions before and also after having been written down.[2] The explanations given in this book are based upon the teachings of Shrii Shrii Anandamurti, the twentieth-century founder of the socio-spiritual organization 'Ananda Marga.'[3] His original thoughts can be found in the book titled: 'A Guide to Human Conduct.'

Anandamurti states in the very first lines of his book that morality is not in itself the final goal of life and that Yama-Niyama are principles designed with an objective beyond themselves, based upon another more deeply underlying recognition of the purpose and value of human life.[4] They are not based upon fear, desire for personal gain in the present or future, or the self-assurance of 'righteousness.' They are, in essence, a recognition of the special human capacity of self-reflection and the desire to convert separation into unity, the impermanence of individuality into the infinite and transcendent. This is the base of the Tantra Yoga propounded by Anandamurti: that there is a universal consciousness reflected within each human being, indeed within the whole creation, and it is the process of experiencing in ever deeper levels this consciousness that gives peace and happiness in life. Parallel to this we are transformed into better people through the amplification of our empathy and the sense of social responsibility that arises through the experience (and not only theory) of interconnectedness.[5] Yama-Niyama are the base upon which this development can occur. They are, in a sense, an ethical formulation 'informed by our 'sense of spiritual potential",[6] a practical reply to the recognition that:

> The impulse to bridge the separation between the small-self and the Spirit has tremendous consequences throughout all the levels and quadrants of human existence. It is as central to to any description of humanity as gravity is to a description of the physical universe.[7]

In order to bridge this separation, or even to develop a clear awareness of this impulse living inside of us and how it affects our lives (more often than not unconsciously), a certain calmness of mind is needed. The principles of Yama-Niyama are a codified explanation of observations as to how the mind works and the attitudes and conduct which will provide the individual with the mental balance needed in order to realize the inspiration of the infinite within their self and in daily life. For this reason they are considered as the foundation of any meditation practice,[8] without which attempts at concentration will be akin to lighting a fire with wet wood: a lot of smoke, little warmth, and increasing frustration. This idea will become clearer as you proceed throughout the book.

Alongside the recognition of the human search for the transcendent, Yama-Niyama incorporates equally a dose of relativism, never forgetting that each and every situation in life is unique. One must apply discernment in every case, not less so but perhaps even more so than if one were to live without any particular code of ethics. Yama-Niyama do not provide the specifics of how one must respond to any given situation, rather the onus is on the individual to reflect, assume responsibility and then decide the best approach to take.[9] What Yama-Niyama do is create the perspective, sensibility and psychic 'design' though which one is able to make decisions fully aware of one's conscious and subconscious intentions.

This act of taking responsibility for one's subconscious is part of what makes Yama-Niyama work, as you will see when you read, for example, the section on 'Satya', which explains the interactions between the conscious and subconscious mind, and how these interactions properly guided create will-power and courage. This psychic strength is in turn the source of mental and emotional balance.

Before going on it is worthwhile becoming familiar with two essential principles of the Tantra-Yoga philosophy of Anandamurti, which are important in and of themselves and also because they are distinct as compared to certain other yogic schools of thought.

First: the world is not an illusion! Unlike Saunkaracarya, who claimed: *'Brahma Satyam Jagat Mithya'*- 'The world is an illusion and only Brahma (infinite consciousness) is truth', and equally unlike Carvaka philosophy which claims that only the material is truth and the abstract does not exist,[10] Anandamurti propounded: *'Brahma Satyam Jagadapi Satyam Ápeksíkam'*- 'Brahma is the absolute truth. This universe is also truth, but a relative one.' [11] Divinity is to be discovered through and within this world and not only beyond it. What is required is not to deny the world but to transform one's experience of it. The existence of the universe is not an illusion, and nor is it to be viewed negatively, as distraction to be rejected as far as possible.

To negate the value of the created world is in itself a rejection of the need for any kind of moral conduct, just as much as hedonism, for example, has no need of ethics. It is also an act of hypocrisy and callousness with the potential of producing a very convoluted interpretation of spirituality, the contradictions of which should be self-apparent.[12] Yama-Niyama, in the very fact of its existence, proclaims loud and clear: 'This world is real! It is ever-changing, but it does exist!' The infinite is there hidden as the essence of all the colourful expressions of life, if you just know where and how to look.

The second notable point of Anandamurti's philosophy, which also relates directly to Yama-Niyama, is the concept of friction as a positive and essential force to growth. Obstacles, he explains, are 'helping forces to reach the goal,' and peace is found in ever increasing degrees through internal and external effort and struggle.[13] Peace of mind, within this scheme of things, is not an anaesthetized state of calm in which one avoids the processing of difficult and transformative life-experiences, nor an escape from the responsibilities of daily life. Rather, one is even encouraged to make special effort to place oneself in challenging situations in order to confront one's fears, contradictions and mental complexes.[14] In this context, what is the meaning of 'mental equilibrium'? It is the state in which one has the strength and composure of mind to maintain a balanced and unbiased perception even when surrounded by disturbing forces. This capacity derives from one's integrity of intent, which in turn derives from the awareness of one's unconscious thought patterns, and of consciously working to integrate into these patterns a sense of univeralism: of interconnectedness and thus of empathy with the entire created world.

The effort of self-reflection and actualization of its results which Yama-Niyama demands produces a kind of mental friction which, as a flour mill grinds wheat into flour, refines the perceptions and emotional state of a person. Each time this effort is made, the mind gains in strength and thus equilibrium, and what begins as a conscious effort is gradually integrated into the subconscious mind to become a natural state of being:

> It cannot be said that the ultimate aim of human life it not to commit theft; what is desirable is that the tendency to commit theft should be eliminated. Not to indulge in falsehood is not the aim of life; what is important is that the tendency of telling lies should be dispelled from one's mind. The sádhaka (spiritual practitioner) starts spiritual practices with the principles of morality, of not indulging in theft or falsehood. The aim of such morality is such a state of oneness with Brahma (infinite consciousness) where no desire is left for theft; and all tendencies of falsehood disappear.[15]

In this sense, Yama-Niyama also serve as a link between the relative and absolute, and a tangential point upon which 'fact' (information derived from the objective world) and 'meaning' have the chance to cordially meet:

A comprehensive account of ethics requires

accepting that they are both *constructed* by humanity and *prior* to humanity… they have both *relative* and *absolute* origins. On the relative side, ethics are socially constructed to help us survive in a contrary universe- they assist the viability of autonomous systems. On the absolute side, ethics are informed by our 'sense' of spiritual potential which first manifests… in the Archetypal mind. It is the level of mind where archetypes such as virtue, beauty, truth, justice and love first differentiate from Spirit and thereby give multiple kinds of meaning to our lives. [16]

Human beings have a tendency to search for absolutes: in beliefs crowned as 'ultimate' truths; in perfect systems; or, equally so, in materialistic reductionism. The problem with this arises not because the desire of the possibility of transcendence is faulty, but because we look in the wrong places and try to convert relativity into this absolute (be it as absolute peace, certainty, etc) that we so desire. This is paradoxical, as by doing so our mental processes and world view are crystallized into dogmas and human creativity is stifled as our unconscious or misunderstood 'thirst for the infinite'[17] is converted into its opposite.

Literature offers no shortage of dystopian novels which vividly demonstrate this point: that human happiness is not to be found in an externally imposed stability and certainty;[18] nor in having our moral and emotional dilemmas solved effortlessly by artificial means; nor even by the simplification of life through the continuous provision of indulgent pleasures.[19]

Inspiration in life comes from the dynamism

produced from the friction of opposing forces and the growth and conversion of the unknown into the known that this produces. That we can learn to appreciate this point and enjoy the process involved in it is made possible through a feeling of love for something greater than one's self being realized within one's self through the process of growth. [20]

The biologist Humberto Maturana, describing how interactions of love effect the evolution of humanity, defines love as 'the domain of those relational behaviours through which the other arises as a legitimate other in coexistence with oneself'[21] and explains that it is love, by creating a space of cooperation, trust and undistorted relationships, that opens the possibility of the liberation of intelligence:

> Love is visionary, not blind, because it liberates intelligence and expands coexistence in cooperation as it expands the domain in which our nervous system operates. Love expands the domain in which our nervous system abstracts coherences from our living.[22]

Love may have many contextual expressions, but its essence is the same, and spiritual love is the 'spontaneous experience of expansion of love' in which 'there is an opening to the total acceptance of the cosmos in unity with oneself.'[23]

What does Yama-Niyama do for us, finally? It creates the balanced state of mind, possible because of the strength gained from clarity of intent, which permits us to develop empathy towards those both known and unknown to us, loving them as expressions of that which is universal within all. Thus every aspect of creation is legitimate and does not need to justify its existential value, but does need be treated according to our best judgement in the given context. Yama-Niyama is the base upon which we become able to expand our love from individual to infinite, through meditation as a spiritual practice and in all endeavours of daily life. This, in my humble understanding and experience, is the motivation behind their design.

YAMA

AHIM'SÁ

Ahim'sá means, in the simplest sense, 'not to inflict harm on others through thought, word or action.[1] 'Thought' here implies mentally, in the realm of intentions, through planning or desiring to do so, whether actualized or not. 'Others' refers not only to human beings but to all living beings, and in this line of thought naturally also includes the creation as a whole, being a composite of living entities and the environment necessary to sustain them.[2]

To properly understand this definition it is first of all necessary to define 'him'sá' (harm), and it is also useful to note the importance of the correlation between 'thought, word and action.' The Yamas are mental attitudes just as much as they are practical actualizations of those attitudes, and therefore always begin in the realm of idea and require a congruence of the inner and outer personality in order to attain their proper meaning and effect. 'Him'sá' refers to any act which stops the further development of a person. This can be in the sense of physical survival, mental or emotional progress, or relating to subtler, inner spiritual sentiments. Although it has at times been defined as such, 'Him'sá' does not mean 'violence' or 'application of force,' as a distinction is made between the concepts of violence and harm. 'Ahim'sá', therefore, should not be defined as 'non-violence' or pacifism. Life in and of itself requires the application of force. This 'force' is not inevitably destructive, but can also be transformational.[3] In a fight between opposing forces, the neutral force is not necessarily the force of good, but quite possibly that of escapism. To defend oneself or another when attacked is bravery, and not to do so cowardice. There is no question here of the intent to harm, but rather of courage in self defence and also of altruism in the case of protecting someone other than oneself.

'Non-violence' as a slogan may serve as a useful political tool, but even then does not automatically imply a moral high-ground placing its followers on a pedestal above criticism. Everything depends, as always, on the context, and there is no universal equation which can automatically deduce the righteousness of any said group or individual in all situations. Violence may at times be justified in order to prevent further harm, though obviously not as something desired, and application of force, for example as circumstantial pressure, also has its place.[4]

Ahim'sá also should not be interpreted in such a way that it makes life impossible. It is not the refusal to kill mosquitoes or to partake in agriculture for fear of killing pests, or a negation (and thus violence towards) one's own body in order to fulfil such ideals.[5] Its purpose is not to produce, in the words of Rabindranath Tagore, a 'piety [that] becomes an unreal abstraction' and (paradoxically) 'deadens the moral sense of an individual.'[6] Like all of Yama-Niyama, ahim'sá is to be understood according to its inner spirit and purpose, which is essentially to cultivate sensitivity and empathy towards others and all forms of life. Ahim'sá is not an injunctive to be conformed with in order to avoid 'bad karma,'[7] or out of fear of future suffering. It should not be followed with this motive, but rather because of the innate value which it carries in and of itself. If one desists in harming others only out fear of the possible negative consequences, although perhaps this may have some social value as long as the control of fear remains (and even in this case it is hardly the preferred base to construct society upon), on a psychological and spiritual level, it means little. In some sense perhaps worse than little, as it produces a kind of hypocrisy in the personality and another problem to be solved in the long-term.   Ahim'sá is not a ritual to be applied mechanically.   It rests upon something much deeper than this, upon some archetypal base of what it means to be human.

What does it mean, in essence, to intend not to harm another, nor to obstruct their progress in any level? It is a recognition of something of ourselves in the other: that we as individuals possess the desire to live and grow, to develop our innate capacity and potential; that this desire exists equally in others; and that the possibility of my own unfolding rests in the expansion of my empathy to include this same intrinsic desire of others as equally valid as my own, and even as part of myself. That, in a sense, one 'becomes all the truer the more he realizes himself in the other.'[8]

Ahim'sá is a recognition of the existential value of life and not only its usefulness. It is the cultivation of subtler human sensibilities and not the utilitarian callousness and cynicism which offers to fill their place, wherein 'he who has no love in him values the gifts of his lover only according to their usefulness.'[9] Expressed in another way:

One thing you might ask yourself is if you believe

each individual is divine. You may say perhaps not, but you certainly act as though you do.[10]

Even when this sentiment is unconscious, or even in denying any concept of 'divinity', generally we do act out such an innate acknowledgement, albeit at times in fits and starts and in a very imperfect way. If we did not, there would be no civilization to speak of. That our civilization is imperfect is a reflection of the fact that we enact this recognition through our imperfections, but not that it is not so, for we continue trying to make it so. When we do not, it reflects back upon us as individuals as psychological and emotional disturbances, or if we become accustomed to it, as a debasement of our sensibilities and perception, and thus a limiting of our intelligence and possibility to growth. On the collective level, when we negate the value of others, see only their mechanical value, or place the value of some above the rest (the collective version of 'oneself' as above everyone else), the result is tyranny and cruelty on a mass scale, of which history has born testimony to countless times.

In Dostoevsky's classic novel, 'Crime and Punishment', the protagonist, Raskolnikov, serves as a kind of symbolic representation of this idea: although intellectually he created every kind of justification for his crime of murder, and emotionally did not experience repentance, yet criminality refused to assimilate and harden into his nature. His actions reflected back on him in the inner psychological level, causing him to become mad. Life disgusted him and all attempts at kindness from others produced a kind of repulsion within him. He sought redemption even whilst rejecting the very idea of it, and even when refusing to feel guilt.[11]

This is what is meant when it was said that ahim'sá rests upon some 'archetypal base of what it means to be human.' It is something we cannot remove from ourselves, not even by actualizing its apparent opposite. In the terminology of Tantra Yoga this can be explained by saying that there is universal consciousness reflected within each human being, and that our innate nature is to seek expansion and to transform into that unconditioned consciousness which is the permanent essence of the self. This is to be done not by negating the world, but by an ever expansive embrace of the entire creation as part of one's self, so that finally there is no other, but instead a sense of unity with all.[12] We seek expansion and harmony and suffer from separation and division, and if we act so as to deny this in another, we are denying something fundamental in our own humanity. The value that we refuse to give to the other expresses itself as an inability to experience that same value in ourselves.

Ahim'sá involves a constant practice of awareness of our attitudes and feelings towards others, which helps to create an undisturbed state of mind receptive to meditation practice, and meditation in turn creates the perception necessary to implement ahim'sá. Meditation works on the subconscious mind, and for this to be possible the conscious mind,[13] full of ever-changing thoughts, sensory experiences etc. has to be brought to calm. The interactions between the subconscious and conscious mind will be explained in more detail in the section about 'satya.' Put simply, actions that go against the principle of ahim'sá cause mental restlessness which makes concentration impossible. Such actions limit one's experiences and perception rather than expand them and are therefore contra to the very purpose of spiritual practice. This applies in respect to physical actions and words as well as to thoughts and desires. In the first stage, such desires will exist, and should be transmuted mentally so that they do not translate into action. In the final stage, they will cease to arise in the mind at all. This is accomplished through a process of channelizing the mind which is known as 'brahmacarya,' the fourth point of the Yamas.

To be properly implemented, Ahim'sá requires a deep reflection about what it means to be a human being, and the meaning of 'helping' and 'harming' within the context of that reflection. The scoldings of a mother to her child, done with love and the spirit of rectification work to a benevolent effect, whereas insincere praise given at the wrong time, perhaps to soothe an uncomfortable situation in the short term, may contribute to produce a distorted, narcissistic personality. What is and is not ahim'sá depends on the context, and the deliberation that it demands has the added benefit of impelling one to continuously reassess the meaning of one's own humanity, and becoming more responsible as a person in the process.

'Harm' may involve something as obvious as causing physical harm through violent abuse; it may be witnessing someone suffering, perhaps an unknown person, and neglecting to help them for the sake of not wanting to complicate one's personal life; or perhaps an act done indirectly, planned by one person but carried out by another; it may be harm by negation, neglecting one's elderly parents, leaving them without company, suffering emotions of abandonment in the final stages of life; harm may be perpetuated in insincere relationships, whereby playing with the emotions of the other for the sake only of personal satisfaction, a cycle of mistrust is born; harm may be mocking someone's sincerity or encouraging their perversion. The list of possibilities are endless. Perhaps one of the first and simplest things to be aware of in this context is how much we are influenced by selfishness. If selfishness and narcissism are there, it is easy to be compelled to harm.

More than physical harm, the deepest afflictions we can cause to another are on the emotional level: manipulations which disturb and confuse the capacity to give and receive love, or which produce cynicism and pessimism in the mind. Such acts can be long-lasting and difficult to undo. They harm by cutting short the natural flow and development of the personality and possibility of a person to comfortably express their full potential as a human being, physically, mentally and spiritually. Often, they create a repeated cycle of harm. The harm is first of all on the receiving end, but also boomerangs back upon the perpetrator, who in the subtle psychological plane is distorting his own emotional well-being. Ahim'sá considers both of these: the effect on the other, and the effect on one's own mind. Who we are is a result of the continuous interaction of our self with the world, a composite of our actions and intentions towards the other. Essentially, there exists nothing that can be considered totally separate from our own self.

On a different note, as through the practice of ahim'sá and meditation one's sense of empathy expands, it also comes to include non-human forms of life. Although it is impossible to live without causing any destruction of life, nonetheless the taking of another creature's life should be avoided as far as possible. There is a difference between the taking of animal life for survival or for the sake only of psychological and sensual satisfaction as food when not really necessary. Ahim'sá, as as part of a spiritual practice, with the goal of developing sensitivity to the value of all life, and knowing that animals also suffer pain and wish to preserve their existence, recommends a vegetarian diet. Aside from the moral aspect, this also has other physical and mental benefits which aid in meditation.[14] In this way, the desire to live and develop that resides within every creature is incorporated into our own sense of self. It is this expansion of sympathy upon which ahim'sá is in essence based.

SATYA

'Satya' is a word without an exact English synonym, but can be defined as 'expression guided by the spirit of benevolence towards others', or 'the use of one's mind and words with the inner spirit of welfare.'[1] It is not 'truthfulness' per se, as often defined, as the word for 'truth' in the sense of 'stating the facts' exactly as they are or as one perceives them to be, is 'rta,' which has a somewhat different implication.[2] Satya could be described as a combination of the inner spirit of honesty, sincerity and integrity applied to speech: words used conscientiously and with benevolent intent.

When satya and rta, benevolence and 'statement of fact', are in agreement, then both can be followed. However, this is not always so and discernment is needed. When there is a conflict between the two, and where rta may cause harm, the spirit of benevolence takes priority.

> That which is a fact, which has really taken place, we call rta... When rta leads to harm, or when it carries the possibility of falsehood, in that case people improve upon rta and make it a fit instrument for promoting welfare. Rta when it leads to welfare is called satya.[3]

Simple examples of situations in which Satya and Rtá are in conflict could include for example, if you were hiding someone in your house to protect them from aggressors, and telling the 'truth' about their presence would result in their harm; or having to reveal news of the tragic and unexpected death of a relative to an elderly person, in which case it would be compassionate to prepare their mind step by step for the news instead of stating outright the facts and causing a mental shock.

Satya, like ahim'sá, does not always give ready-made answers. It recognizes that human beings possess the capacity for rationality and discernment, and demands that we develop and use them.[4] It requires at times a confrontation with one's own conscience and motivations in order to be meaningful. To understand the inner import of satya as an ethical and spiritual practice, it is useful to understand how it effects the interactions between the conscious, subconscious and unconscious minds, and the connection this has to the development of will-power, self-confidence, and personal integrity, or what in Sanskrit is know as 'rjuta,' or 'straightforwardness.'

Unlike western psychology, which still lacks any precise definition of what 'mind' is, meditation practices are based upon a systematized conceptualization of the mind and its functions. These observations include many very meticulous and insightful descriptions about the nature of perception, consciousness, and interactions between subjective and objective realities. [5]

Basically, the mind or mental functions are divided into various levels, each responsible for a certain kind of perception. These levels can be called the 'conscious', 'subconscious' and 'unconscious' layers of the mind. Although there are parallels, the terms are used differently to in other schools of Western psychology. More accurately and to avoid confusion, these layers can also be described as the 'crude', 'subtle' and 'causal' minds, or for the sake of easier conceptualization, as the 'pre-personal', 'personal', and 'trans-personal' minds. Beyond these levels lies pure, unconditioned and unchanging consciousness, the state which meditation practices seek finally to embody.[6]

The conscious mind is that part of the mind which is always intimately connected with the objective, material world, and with the physical body. It receives and takes the forms of external objects and sensory perceptions and also deals with physical impulses and instincts. As the external world is ever-changing, so to the conscious mind is always restless. It is actually in some ways the least 'aware' or 'conscious' of all the layers of mind. In Sanskrit this layer is called the 'kamamaya kosa', 'kama' meaning mental tendencies relating to the physical world.[7]

The subconscious or subtle mind in Sanskrit is known as the 'manomaya kosa.' 'Man' literally means 'mind,' and includes within its scope capacities such as rationality, abstraction and symbolisation, self-reflection, and most of the subjective, inner emotional world of a human being.[8] While the conscious mind acts out impulses or habituated behaviours without awareness of their origins or motives, the source of these behaviours and the deeper emotional processes behind them lies in the subconscious mind. The possibility of understanding, guiding and transforming them also lies in the subconscious. Meditation, and all of Yama-Niyama, work upon the subconscious and subjective inner world, and from there, create a transformation in our interactions with and experience of objective reality. Until we develop a relationship of familiarity with the subconscious, we are slaves to the restlessness of the mind and body. To a point, this can be compared with the Jungian Psycholgy when it speaks of the integration of the 'unconscious' processes into the personality. The yogic descriptions, however, are rather more specific and systematic in their definitions.

Aside from its significance as the realm of our inner world and therefore our functioning as an emotional, rational and reflective entity, the importance of the subconscious also lies in its role as a link between the conscious and the unconscious minds. Normally, the conscious mind is engaged in direct interactions with the physical world, whereas the subconscious mind interacts with and through the conscious mind. The processes of self-reflection, meditation and Yama-Niyama add a new dimension to this interaction. The 'unconscious mind', more correctly called the 'causal mind', is trans-personal in nature. It is not unique to the individual, although the perceptions gained from the unconscious do depend to an extent on the individual tendencies of the subconscious. The causal mind is further divided into three levels, which are quite abstract but can be described as the 'intuitive', 'archetypal' and 'universal' minds.[9] In the same way that the conscious receives input from the subconscious, the subconscious is linked to the causal or unconscious, and the unconscious to pure consciousness, the unchanging and eternal essence of the self. Within this scheme, it is also understood that the universe is a creation formed from pure consciousness, as an 'internal thought process' of that consciousness. When the individual mind, through its link with the subconscious, accesses the unconscious, it is entering this 'trans-personal' cosmic mind, a non-sensory source of wisdom and creative processes.

Meditation, aided by Yama-Niyama, stills the conscious mind until such a point that it merges into the subconscious. A clear vision of the subconscious is thus gained. The unconscious, normally having an almost entirely inactive role in the psyche, begins to be 'lit-up' by the clarity or light then present in the subconscious. This is not to say that it was a dark place, but only that it was until then unknown. It is as if the subconscious were a lower room connected to an upper one by an opaque wall. As long as the lower floor was only dimly lit, the upper one was completely invisible. When the lower floor is sufficiently and brightly lit up, one can see and gain knowledge of the upper one. When the subconscious becomes totally calm, it merges into the unconscious, and so on, ever closer to the universal soul which is the essence of the self.

This process produces a modification in the normal patterns and activities of the mind. Instead of only being an interchange between the external world, the conscious and the subconscious, the subconscious begins receiving another kind of inspiration, an expanded perception and vision, from the unconscious. This creates a change in the subconscious, and thus in the source of all our emotional expressions, intellectual processes, thoughts, and experience. As these transform, our desires and their actualizations also change, and the physical body, glands, hormonal processes that create the emotions, and nerves adjust accordingly.[10] A world view defined by separation, isolation, selfishness, etc. transforms into one defined by the unity of interconnectedness, harmony, empathy and insight. In the practical level, this results in self-confidence, courage, will-power and selflessness. It also creates a feeling of hope in the deepest sense of the term.

How is this connected to the practise of satya? In Eastern cosmology, the mind as well as the universe are described as a 'spectrum of waves' whose 'wave-length decreases from subtler to cruder levels.'[11] Matter is made up of the densest waves, with the most curvatures, whereas mind is increasingly subtler depending on the level of awareness, and pure consciousness has no vibration, it is as though a perfectly straight line, beyond all conditioning and relativity. Meditation can be described as the process of straightening the waves of the conditioned mind until they merge with unconditioned consciousness.[12] Satya facilitates this process, as it removes the convolutions of the thought processes and replaces them with a clarity which allows one to surpass the limiting emotional structures and conditioning of the self. Satya is the applied side of meditation, the practical expression of this straightening of the mental vibrations:

> ...the ideal of supreme freedom of consciousness... is not merely intellectual or emotional, it has an ethical basis and it must be translated into action.[13]

Speech is the external expression of thought, and satya is therefore first of all a state of mind and then an external actualization of that state. Hypocrisy describes the incongruence between ones thoughts and intentions, and words or actions. This incongruence or lack of internal honesty, especially when it become habitual and integrated into the personality, is contrary to the expansion of mind which meditation seeks. It disturbs the mind and inhibits access to the subconscious. If the subconscious mind cannot be accessed, meditation is impossible.

To take an example from popular literature, J.R.R. Tolkien in the 'Lord of the Rings' has provided a perfect archetype of this incongruence and lack of satya through the character of Saruman. Saruman, although of vast knowledge, possessed certain contradictions in his personality which led to his ultimate downfall. Most notably, he possessed the 'power of his voice.' He knew how to use words to manipulate and twist the thoughts and decisions of others, something akin to a modern politician.[14] The power of his rhetoric, Tolkien himself clarifies, was no magic spell, but rather lay in his capacity of persuasion:

> Saruman's voice was not hypnotic but persuasive. Those who listened to him were not in danger of falling into a trance, but of agreeing with his arguments, while fully awake. It was always open to one to reject, by free will and reason, both his voice while speaking and its after-impressions. Saruman corrupted the reasoning powers.[15]

As much as he used this power over others, he distorted his own inner vision, and it could be concluded that because of this was also manipulated, leading to his final and utterly humiliating end. This is in contrast to his contemporary, Gandalf, who although skilled in diplomacy and ever-careful in his choice of words, never lost his clarity of mind in the traps of false intentions. The rhetoric of each was an expression of the inner workings of their minds, which lead to the downfall of one and the success of the other.[16]

'Rjuta,' as already mentioned, is a Sanskrit word which can be translated as 'straightforwardness.' Satya creates this Rjuta, or inner straightforwardness, unravelling the convolutions of the mind. Knowing that one has not done wrong nor intends to do so, the mind develops strength, courage, and mental composure.[17] One becomes self-confident in a way that does not depend on external forces of encouragement. The firmest base of will-power and self-esteem is the clarity and autonomy of personality created by following satya. The opposite is also true: internal contradictions affect the will, and the mind and nervous system become weakened and depressed, loosing the motivation to face the challenges of life. Hope is one tendency which human beings cannot live without. Not so much hope in the sense of 'something good will happen' or that 'my wishes will be fulfilled', but rather in the sense of possibility of unfolding, of being able to discover and fulfil one's potential, practically but even more importantly internally: the hope of ever discovering the depths of the self and the essence of life. When hope is destroyed, life has no meaning. The sustaining and fulfilment of hope rests in satya, as that which, as already explained, inspires the personality with integrity, confidence and the will to overcome obstacles using the force of benevolence.

Philosophically, the word 'satya' is also used to

refer to universal consciousness, which has been described as 'the essence of satya.' It is there that there are no contradictions, no discordance of opposites, but only the perfectly straight flow of unconditioned awareness.[18] The practical side of satya deals with the objective world, but internally, its seeks its own essence, the satya of pure consciousness.

<u>ASTEYA</u>

Asteya means 'not to take possession of that which belongs to another', nor to cultivate the mental desire to do so. It is 'non-stealing' in both thought and practice.[1]

The reasons behind this point are much the same as those given regarding satya: actions and desires contra to asteya create a labyrinth of mental complications and as a result restlessness in the subconscious mind. The person who steals cannot be straightforward or follow satya, as they must resort to dishonesty in order to hide their behaviour, and this dishonesty in turn produces its own psychological results. In addition, the desire for the property of others can easily create unhealthy material obsessions and produce negative patterns of jealousy, resentment, etc.

Like ahim'sá and satya, asteya also begins in the mind. Not to steal out of fear of punishment is not asteya. This only creates a dual personality, devoid of satya and also of simplicity. Asteya means not to steal out of principle, and also not to desire to do so. The psychological background to one's actions is what counts most.

Asteya is divided into two categories. The first is the actual physical theft of any object, and the second involves indirectly depriving someone through cheating, manipulation or corruption.[2] When one steals from another, it is not only a physical object that is concerned. One does not know the work that was involved by the other person in earning the stolen object, what it was needed for, or the sentimental

importance it may have held. Anyone who has had
something of even minimal personal value stolen from
them will understand the feeling of betrayal involved.

A 'Robin Hood' mentality is also not compatible
with asteya. Even if the property of another was gained
undeservedly, or due to unjust socio-economic
structures, this does not give one the right to steal. If
the problem lies in badly designed social systems, in
corruption, or faulty economic planning, then an effort
must be made to solve the source of these problems in
order to facilitate proper re-distribution of wealth,
wages, and opportunities. This takes thought, effort
and struggle. Desiring and dishonestly acquiring the
property of another in this context, or 'robbing from the
rich to give to the poor,' falls somewhere between being
'an easy way out' of what are deeper, systemic
problems, the continuation of a negative cycle, or a
mental trick justifying opportunism. It is not beneficial
psychologically to the individual, and nor is it a proper
mentality upon which to attempt to build a better social
system.[3]

Albeit in a slightly different context, Anandamurti
amplifies upon this point in other texts,[4] explaining that
according to the essence of spirituality, the material
world is never the true property of anybody, and one
has only the right to safe-guard and use it. It is the
responsibility of human society to find the best way to
employ and divide the world's resources for the benefit
of all. Human beings have a natural attachment to their
property, and the desire to earn according to their
efforts and merit, which should always be recognized.
At the same time the inner spirit of 'ownership' as
being not to 'own' something per se but to have the

responsibility to care for and utilize any specific thing towards a constructive outcome should be cultivated.[5]

The second aspect of asteya describes acts of cheating: not paying someone for services provided; travelling by public transport without a ticket; claiming benefits which one is not entitled to; or the misuse of intellectual property. Asteya is in many ways an extension of satya in relation to acquisition of property and wealth. The spirit of asteya, combined with satya, can also be extended to abstract acquisitions. In this way, for example, obtaining influence, power, or employment undeserved, (and thus depriving another of the same) through false qualifications, nepotism or bribery goes against not only asteya, but also satya and ahim'sá. Although the implications of asteya are somewhat simpler that those of satya and ahim'sá, it too requires self-reflection and a sense of responsibility as to the consequences of one's actions and desires.

BRAHMACARYA

Brahmacarya refers to the constant awareness of Brahma (divine consciousness) in all that one does and all the entities and objects that one deals with. As already explained, the base of yoga, and from the specific perspective of this book, of tantric meditation practices, is the effort to produce an expansion of individual consciousness, directed towards the attainment of a state of unconditioned, universal consciousness. This consciousness is considered to be the essence of the self and also the essential substance of creation, and therefore, as the individual experiences and identifies with it in ever-increasing degrees, all that is apparently external is embraced as a part one's own existence. Isolation and separation are replaced by a pervasive sense of unity. The 'Brahma' of brahmacarya refers to this universal consciousness. Brahmacarya is the awareness of the essence of things instead of only their superficial appearance, through which all the actions and objects of everyday life find their place as part of the inner spiritual search.

> ... (its) doctrine is transcendence through active participation... the finite is a symbol of the infinite. The infinite stamps its seal onto its own nature replete with all the possible forms of the infinite.[1]

This idea has been expressed well by Mark Dyczkowski in his comparison between the world-view of Kashmiri Saivism (a form of tantra) and Vedanta:

The Shaiva method is one of ever widening inclusion of phenomena mistakenly thought to be outside the absolute. The Vedantin, on the other hand, seeks to understand the nature of the absolute by excluding (nisedha) everything which does not conform to the criterion of absoluteness, until all that remains is the unqualified Brahma. The Saiva's approach is one of affirmation and the Vedantin's one of negation.[2]

Brahmacarya is an expression of the first method, which embraces all the varied expressions of the world as fundamentally divine. This refers as much to objects and actions as to the subjective experiences connected to and produced by them. In this context, the 'Vijinana Bhairava Tantra,' makes an interesting observation, explaining how any intense experience, if traced back to its essential source, can be used to benefit spiritual awareness. During intense emotional experiences, the mind becomes totally focused and absorbed in what is happening. Such moments, whether joyful or painful, are ephemeral. The mind not grasping their essence, in the case of joyful experiences, desires the permanence of something which is by nature limited, and as a result remains restless. If the experiences are extremely painful, one tries to reject them, also without comprehending their inner meaning. If however one is able to transcend the limited perception of one's thought constructs and observe the inner (and eternal) essence of such experiences, and at the same time be attentive to the way in which which the mind becomes absorbed in any feeling, this understanding of the mental process involved can be utilized in spiritual practice, and the same intensity and process of absorption can be applied to the one ideation that is beyond the conditioning of relativity: 'I am Brahma,' the pervasive universal consciousness.[3]

Anandamurti echoes a similar sentiment when he says that a spiritual practitioner should not destroy the tendencies of the mind, but instead learn how to utilize them to their benefit.[4] Brahmacarya rests within this context and approach to spirituality, applying it to all interactions and work of daily life, from the most mundane moments to the most exceptional ones.

Before explaining further the application and benefits of brahmacarya, it is worthwhile to be aware of some misinterpretations of the term, which can be found in numerous texts and commentaries. It is very common to find brahmacarya translated as 'celibacy,' which is then sometimes re-interpreted in a variety of different ways in order to make it a little more palatable to the modern yoga student.[5] This 're-definition' is hardly necessary, since the etymology of brahmacarya contains no mention of sexuality or celibacy. Although it could be said that 'brahmacarya', properly defined as the constant awareness of Brahma, may aid in integrating sexuality into one's life in a balanced way, or vice versa, that a sexuality properly integrated and understood will facilitate the practice of brahmacarya, this is not the definition nor focus of the term itself. Anandamurti goes so far as to say that brahmacarya defined as celibacy was an invention of a certain class of supposedly 'religious' people at a historical junction when they attempted to impose their control and superiority over the masses of society. Defining the term in such a way imposed a complex of spiritual inferiority on the general population, and opened the path to exploitation:[6]

This peculiar interpretation of brahmacarya may contain anything and everything save except satya. Hence there is no dharma or brahma in it.[7]

Certainly there is a place for celibate life for those with the inclination to it. It is a choice well-suited to someone who wants to dedicate themselves specifically to some special work or study that will be of benefit to society, or who simply has other interests. In this case celibacy is not the focus in and of itself but a means to a certain end, which is the benefit of the freedom of exclusive concentration born of commitment to a cause, and the space then created to dedicate one's energy to that goal.[8] The commitment of a well-planned family life is also ideal for spiritual practices, providing the stimulating challenge of balancing service to one's family and to society in general.[9]

Of course, brahmacarya even in its correct definition will touch indirectly on how sexuality is incorporated into individual and collective life. In the same way, so will ahimsa and satya, just as they connect to almost any other aspect of the psyche. That one's predominating tendency is to view the opposite gender as an object for sexual gratification, or that this is the exclusive thought that comes to mind before any other quality that a person may have, obviously is not in accordance with the spirit of brahmacarya. In the same line, sexuality used as a form of emotional manipulation or blackmail, be it consciously or unconsciously, does not sit well with satya. Regarding ahim'sá, there are the traumatic psychological consequences of abuse; the effects of economic interests based upon coercion or perversion; or irresponsible relationships as the source of cynicism and loss of trust in human interactions due to lack of sincerity or depth of reflection. In this sense, for the attentive, focused and empathetic state of mind required for meditation, yes, it is recommended that this aspect of the human personality is integrated into daily life in a sensible way according to the context and the individual, so that it produces something constructive and not destructive: love, compassion and growth and not narcissism. Perhaps the defining point here is that however this is done, it should be a decision taken with awareness and a sense of responsibility.

Brahmacarya is an internal attitude applied externally. During meditation, one guides the mind in a particular style so as to experience in ever increasing degrees the unconditioned awareness which is the essence of the self: the ideation that 'I am Brahma.' Brahmacarya then applies this to the external world, ie. 'this world is also Brahma'.[10] The mind, having a steady reference point, is able to maintain a broad and balanced perspective without becoming distracted or dispersed even whilst moving between daily tasks and material necessities.

Psychologically speaking, this is a subtle and effective way of channelizing the flow of the mind. The mind, with all its feelings, hopes, and desires, is like a river which if blocked, at some point will overflow. It cannot be controlled only by external restrictions or ideals which have not been properly internalized, and which will eventually result in suppression and unhealthy mental reactions. At the same time, a river without the two banks which guide and apparently limit it, cannot move ahead. It ceases to be a river and becomes a stagnant pool. 'Freedom' without a goal, or in the name of ego-centrism or escapism from the challenges and existential questions of human life is like saying that we have 'infinite freedom to fetter ourselves,' not realizing that 'the fettering ends the freedom.'[11] In the river of the mind we cannot build dams, but nor can we remove its banks, apparent limitations which in fact provide the current with its direction and dynamism:

> Our life, like a river, strikes its banks not to find itself closed in by them, but to realise anew every moment that it has its unending opening towards the sea.[12]

Our work then, is to construct the river banks of the mind in such a way as to guide the water so that it can flow easily and freely towards a deepening of the self and a refining of our human sensibilities: to transform the very structures of the subconscious so that these changes becomes a permanent and spontaneous expression of that which we truly are, or have truly to become. Or in the words of the Persian poet Sohrab Sepehri:

> Like a river flowing let us be...
> ...Let us constantly create our own two borders,
> and every minute liberate them. Let us go, let us go,
> whispering of the absence of borders.[13]

Brahmacarya serves as the guiding principle to direct the river: a constant search for and recognition of the depths of meaning in all that we do and all that surrounds us. Our responsibilities, both pleasurable and painful, and at times intensely so, become part of this recognition, and searching for the essence of themselves, surpass themselves; we enjoy the material world not with the desire of possessing it, but for what it is, for the questions it poses us and the possibilities it whispers of; love seeks its own source, and we love not to possess but for the infinite that is within the person that we love, with love serving as a catalyst for its own unfolding. We can plant a garden, clean a house, prepare a meal, with this same idea working in our minds. Pain and pleasure are not suppressed or rejected, but understood as part of the necessary friction in the river of the mind which helps to move the waters ahead and take their rightful place in reference to a deeper vision of life.[14] Remembering brahmacarya, we also remember ahim'sá, satya, asteya and aparigraha.

Brahmacarya serves as the subterranean flow of inspiration for the other Yamas, and provides a touch of the eternal amidst the world of relativity which ethics deals with. It begins as a kind of auto-suggestion, an attempt at awareness, which as we proceed on the spiritual path and grow as human beings, transforms step-by-step into an actual state of being.

APARIGRAHA

Aparigraha is the spirit of 'simple living,' of using material resources in accordance with and in proportion to one's actual needs and not in excess.[1] Where brahmacarya is the awareness of one's inner, subjective approach to the material world, aparigraha refers to the attitude of self-restraint in regards to the actual practical use and possession of material objects. In the collective level, it is an acknowledgement of the fact that material resources are limited and that unrestrained use or irrational distribution of these resources by individuals or any one social group or country has ethical and practical repercussions for the rest of society as well as the natural environment. On the psychological level, aparigraha recognizes that although human beings require a certain level of material comfort in order to fully develop their capacity and potential and also to share that capacity with society, material comfort in itself is not the goal of life nor the ultimate source of inner-satisfaction. To the contrary, the attempt to supply material answers to emotional and spiritual questions, confusing the search for meaning and growth with an incessant search for pleasure, is a source of mental restlessness on the individual level and social injustice collectively.

Aparigraha is the external manifestation of santos'a, or mental contentment, one of the niyamas which will be discussed later. It is an expression of the mental balance which derives from knowing, rationally and consciously, what and how much one actually needs on the material plane, and also the limits of the happiness that material possessions can provide, and that as human beings we are more than just our physical wants.

Aparigraha should not be conceived as a denial of physical necessities, but as a search for balance. Here an apt comparison has been made with the interplay of the body's dual set of desires: on one hand the impulse to self-centred physical gratification and on the other the desire for health. This search for health has been described as:

> '...the desire of our physical system as a whole, of which we are usually unconscious... has no concern with the fulfilment of immediate bodily desires, it goes beyond the present time. It is the principle of wholeness, it links our life with its past and its future and maintains the unity of its parts. He who is wise know it, and makes his other physical wishes harmonise with it.'[2]

The same can be applied to the social body, as an organism in which we as individuals are the cells, and in this context, just as one seeks health in the balance of individual physical desires and needs, 'he who is wise tries to harmonise the wishes which seek for self-gratification with the wish for social good,'[3] and in this way, the mind is able first of all to know itself and its own thought patterns and psychological processes through self-reflection and restraint, and then to grow beyond them. Here the same comparison already given in the explanation of brahmacarya, of the mind as a river and the apparent limitations of the banks being in fact the river's impulse to movement, can also be applied. The other option is of human life as a 'tragedy' which 'consists in vain attempts to stretch the limits of things that can never be unlimited,'[4] instead of coming to understand their true nature and purpose, and the resulting dissatisfaction of such an endeavour.

Aparigraha, like all of Yama-Niyama, is based upon the recognition of the relativity of our lived experiences, even as that relativity seeks the experience of an unconditioned universal principle. The material needs of each person are different, just as each physical body's requirements for food vary depending on the body mass, activities, and climate. These needs also depend on each individual's conception of happiness and comfort. An intellectually minded person, working as a university professor requires books and academic materials in order to complete his work and feel fulfilled. For another, such things may appear absolutely superfluous. A sculptor needs space and materials with which to work, a gardener earth, tools and seeds. Everyone needs food, housing, clothing and medical care, but no one needs designer labels, or land and property beyond their house to live in, work or grow food upon. The underlying spirit of aparigraha is that as inner-satisfaction deepens, one's material needs naturally decrease, and in addition to this natural occurrence, a conscious effort should also be made to reduce them out of empathy and the altruistic desire to then offer what one no longer needs or the time and energy which was previously focused in fulfilling material desires, for the benefit of society at large.

There is another Sanskrit term, 'vaerágya', which evokes this same spirit. Vaerágya has at times been interpreted to mean renunciation from the world and retreat into a life of self-denial and austerity for some imagined spiritual gain. Anandamurti clarifies this and claims that 'it only means to attempt to understand the proper use of things and to use them correctly,'[5] or in other words, the act of balanced perception which prevents the mind from being affected by an excessive or irrational attraction or repulsion towards the said object:

> This right use of a thing is vaerágya. Right use of anything within the idea of vaerágya does not make one's mind a slave to constant longing for the object... (by) not being constantly attracted by crude things, one's mind becomes subtle...[6]

Vaeragya is reached through the act of conscious discernment and awareness, known as viveka:

> The same thing by change in its use can become good or evil, and discrimination between the two is viveka. It is with discrimination (viveka) only that the mind can determine the goodness or evil in a thing or in its uses. Viveka is, therefore, necessary for following vaerágya...[7]

The inner contentment and equilibrium bought about through spiritual practice, aided by vaeragya and viveka (which are also developed and refined through the self-awareness gained in meditation, and in turn assist meditation practice), is expressed practically as aparigraha: a common-sense use of material assets based in what Anandamurti described as the 'maximum utilization and rational distribution of resources for the benefit of all.'[8] Here aparigraha shifts from being an individual attitude and becomes additionally an approach to be reflected in social and economic life. Yama-Niyama are, as much as a base upon which spiritual practice becomes possible, also the fundamentals upon which a healthy society can be constructed. A functioning society depends on the cooperation of its members, and this cooperation depends in turn on a well-thought out code of ethics which supports the development of empathy, mutual trust, and healthy collaboration, and which seeks to build an environment in which the diverse expressions of humanity can thrive and discover the best of themselves. Here the question also then becomes how to structure an efficient and also ethical economy which supports a rational distribution of resources, and whose institutions and businesses, through the inherent nature of their design, foster a cooperative spirit and sense of collective responsibility. Such a design should encourage ethical behaviour, but would also depend on it in order to function, treating economics, human relationships and culture as interlinked aspects of each other.[9] Thus aparigraha begins as a personal endeavour, and leads by its very nature to practical questions about collective life and socio-economic systems.

NIYAMA

<u>SHAOCA</u>

Shaoca (pronounced 'shao-cha') means 'purity' or 'cleanliness.'[1] This has an external as well as internal aspect, and is in used in reference to the body, mind and environment. As the Niyamas are basically internal psychological attitudes or processes, the focus of shaoca is internal and mental, with the external aspects being facilitators of the desired internal state.

Let us assume, as a general premise and without going into details, that our perception of events and emotional experience of them is coloured by a combination of our subconscious mental processes, which are supported by habits ingrained in the hormonal and nervous systems; by past and present experiences; and by stimuli received from the external environment. The yogic world-view also proposes that a certain part of all these are made up of impressions of past actions (from current and previous lives) waiting to express themselves. These are known and 'samskaras,' and create the base of our personality and psychological orientation, which together with out free-will and other environmental influences, create each individual's personality.[2] All of these influences, past and present, internal and external, physical and psychic, combine to create our unique and conditioned subjective experience of life. To give a simple visual example, imagine the mind as a perfectly smooth, round ball of dough. Every action that we perform or imagine, and every stimuli the body and mind receives, creates an impression on the mind, the same way that a ball of dough, when poked by a finger, changes its form. These impressions (samskaras) are the conditioning or 'complexes' of the mind, and because of them we experience the world as we do. The samskaras long to express themselves so that the mind can return to its original form and the unconditioned experience of the self that this invokes.[3]

Shaoca, in this context, relates to what we allow into our minds, considering the mental impression and therefore emotional and character traits which will be produced as a result. Our mental complexes, be they of shame, fear, selfishness, or whatever other form they may take, create distortions in the mind which are then reflected in one's behaviour towards others and the world.[4] The same applies to any kind of emotional impulses or self-centred desires acted upon without awareness or guidance of the conscience. Shoaca, 'mental cleanliness,' is the act of being conscious of and taking responsibility for what we allow into our minds and the psychological patterns we encourage, and also the act of 'cleaning up' whatever has already found a home in the messy room of the inner-self.

To better understand the dynamics of shaoca, it can be divided into four parts: 'external-physical,' 'internal-physical,' external-psychic,' and 'internal-psychic.'

'External-physical' shaoca refers to the effort to maintain the body and natural environment in such a way as to create a state of physical and mental ease conducive to proper psychic development and magnanimity of mind, instead of mental agitation and self-centredness, which make one unable to sympathise with the feelings of others and therefore increase the possibility of inflicting harm, knowingly or not. In this regard, yoga is very practical and offers a wide array of advice about the maintenance of the physical body, with especial focus on the nervous and hormonal systems, recognizing that even when one consciously desires to to good, sometimes the body and glands themselves work contra to this desire.[5] One of the primary functions of the physical practices of yoga is to help minimise this conflict. Yoga postures, or asanas, are designed to work specifically with the glandular, lymphatic and nervous systems to create a harmonious functioning of the body, mind and emotions. The same can be said of yogic advice about regular bathing, for example, and other practices regarding physical cleanliness.[6]

This idea can also be explained in another way through the conceptualization of the cakra system as an emotional map of the body in relation the glands. Here the idea is that each of the cakras is connected with certain psychic tendencies, known as 'vrtiis.' The muladhara cakra, located in the base of the spine, relates to the four basic currents of human desire: physical, psychic, psycho-spiritual and spiritual (kama, artha, dharma and moksa). These are all essential aspects of human existence, however for each of them to find its proper place, the physical should be guided by the psychic, and the psychic by the spiritual. If the entire mental energy gravitates around physical desires, then the subtler human sensibilities will not have the chance to develop. On the other hand, when the physical desires are guided by the mind, they will be able to incorporate themselves into the entire scheme of things in a constructive way. In this case, existing in connection with subtle human emotions, empathy and affection, instead of only as blind instinctual forces of survival, they take on new forms and find their proper place within human culture.

The svadhistana cakra, located above the muladhara but below the navel, is connected to self-centred tendencies such as cruelty, belittlement, or lack of common-sense. The manipura cakra, located at the navel point, is dynamic in nature and is responsible for maintaining a balance between the two lower and two higher cakras. It also contains self-centred and limiting tendencies such as fear, shyness or revulsion, but these are more emotional and less purely instinctual.[7] When the lower cakras and related glands are over-stimulated or agitated, the manipura will be unable to manage its moderator's role, the tendencies of the lower cakras will take over, and selfishness and impulsive gratification will become the dominating forces. If the glands relating to the lower cakras are functioning in a balanced way, the manipura will be guided by the higher cakras, the anahata and vishuddha, and the flow of psychic tendencies will become increasingly magnanimous and altruistic. In this case all the functions of the human body and tendencies of the mind will start to find their appropriate place in individual life and further psychic and spiritual development will proceed naturally, step by step. 'External-physical' shaoca then is the effort to care for the body and endocrine system, through an understanding of the body's interrelation with the mind, in order to regulate it in the simplest and most natural way possible.

Although this explanation of the cakra system is not essential for understanding the external aspects of shaoca, it is an interesting and insightful addition to the point. Something similar applies to 'internal-physical' shaoca. 'Internal-physical' shaoca refers to the yogic science of food, and the idea that what we eat, which in turn forms all the cells of the body and the hormones produced by the glands, also has an effect on one's emotional state and psychic sensibilities, and on the capacity to focus and deepen meditation practices. Thus food should be selected in such a way that it facilitates the state of mind conducive to the real shaoca, which is psychic.[8]

'External psychic' shaoca refers to what one sees and accepts into the mind from the external world. It means to guide the senses so that they assimilate what is helpful to one's mental progress and emotional development, and form the habit of avoiding that which would be detrimental. The idea here is that whatever is taken into the mind on a regular basis creates ingrained psychic or neurological patterns which repeat themselves even when the given stimuli are not physically present, weakening the will-power and making such habits every time more difficult to resist. The idea of shaoca here is to maintain the 'cleanliness' of the mind, through conscious training and awareness of what one wants to assimilate into one's thoughts, instead of accepting whatever comes one's way and later having to clean up the mess. In the beginning this takes some effort, but then slowly becomes a natural process as new psychic patterns are created and enforced.   Such a practice also aids in spiritual meditation as it helps to develop strength and focus of mind.

Apart from dealing with the habit-forming nature of the mind, external-psychic shaoca is also indirectly connected to the idea of developing a mental focus based on the capacity to find value and take pleasure in the effort towards constructive desires and creative effort, instead of the attraction to immediate gratification which does not require the development of any sort of depth of character, and offers 'rewards' which do not demand any sort of responsibility or empathy on the part of the receiver. In the latter case, human creative energy is wasted, and one never becomes aware of one's own motivations and thought-processes, nor of what one really desires from life and the means of creating the conditions to achieve it. Evoking Aldous Huxley's 'Brave New World', one becomes a slave to the instant and superficial gratification of the senses without any purpose beyond the gratification itself, remaining in an infantile emotional state, and is easily manipulated and controlled, a captive of one's own mind as well as the sway of external influences.[9]

The first three aspects of shaoca lead to the third, 'internal-psychic' shaoca. This is the effort to maintain pure intentions internally, and to replace selfishness with magnanimity. It is partly achieved through the awareness and channelization of ones thoughts, partly through one's interactions with others, and also through the process of meditation itself.

Here the practice of shaoca can be compared to that of cleaning a window, outside of which lies an expansive and fascinating view. When it is dirty, the view will be obstructed. The subtly changing patterns of light, the sunrise, sunset or the clear warmth of the daylight sun, will not reach our retinas in quite the same way. Or perhaps, imagine seeing the world through eyes opaqued by cataracts. Shaoca is the cleaning of the window, which needs to be done regularly, so as to gain a perfect view of the landscape: the cleaning of the mind in order to see the world as it is, penetrating ever deeper into its essential nature, and not as our mental complexes and conditioning reflected back on us.

A simple technique to facilitate this 'mental cleaning' is to take up an idea of the opposite nature whenever an unwanted or negative tendency appears in the mind, and to use one's will-power to follow that idea. In this way, the negative tendency is neutralized and strength of mind also develops. For example, if you feel jealous of someone else's happiness, counter it with the idea of friendliness; if you feel envy about someone's progress, counter it by encouraging them to move ahead. Begin by countering the negative idea mentally, and then, as far as possible, actualize this mental effort in practice. Where there is selfishness in the mind, make an effort to expand it into universalism, by service without the desire for recognition, which will probably go unrecognised and without praise from others. There is a shloka from the Buddha Vanii which advises:

Akkodhena jine kodhaṁ asádhuṁ sádhuná jine
Jine kadariiyaṁ dánena sattyena aliikavádinam.

Overcome anger by patience, overcome dishonesty by honesty, overcome greed by generosity, overcome falsehood by truth.[10]

This idea, applied internally and directed towards the

tendencies of one's own mind, and combined with a meditation practice which seeks for expansion of the mind from a self-centred to a universalistic approach to life, forms a firm base for internal-psychic shaoca. Or, in the words of P. R. Sarkar:

> When the flow of the mind is not impeded by selfishness, narrowness, and superstitions that alone is mukti (liberation).[11]

Shaoca is this effort to remove selfishness, narrowness and dogma from the mind, and through this process we can begin to understand the real meaning and experience of 'freedom' and of 'mukti' or 'spiritual liberation.'

SANTOS'A

Santos'a is another word without an exact English translation. Although it can be translated as 'contentment', more explanation is needed in order to understand its precise meaning. 'Tos'a' means 'contentment' in the sense of the 'state of mental ease' felt after having fulfilled one's desire for a particular object or experience. Santos'a can be defined as 'thorough contentment', or 'a state of proper/complete internal ease.'[1] The question then is what is the difference between these two? To grasp this, it is first of all necessary to also know the difference between two more terms: 'sukha' and 'ananda.' Sukha means 'happiness,' in reference to the pleasure that one feels when experiencing a situation in accordance with one's particular psychological inclination, or expressed in another way, in accordance with one's 'samskaras' or mental tendencies resulting from the impressions formed from past actions seeking to be expressed, as explained in the previous chapter.[2] Like everything of the relative world, 'sukha' is transitory and also has its opposite expression, 'dukha,' pain and suffering. Life is a continuous dance in the spaces between and combinations of these pairs of opposites. It should also be noted that this 'sukha' does not necessarily imply something constructive or positive per se. What is considered pleasurable by one may be considered equally unpleasant or tiresome to another, and of course our inclinations may change with time, depending on circumstantial or internal changes in the individual.

Sukha may even refer to happiness derived from destructive habits, sadistic or narcissistic tendencies, etc. Tos'a is the contentment gained through a pleasurable experience in accordance with one's likings, when one feels satiated with the given experience. To give a simple example: you desire to eat chocolate. Until you can fulfil this desire, the mind remains unsatisfied. On obtaining a certain amount of chocolate and consuming it, the desire is relieved and you are contented. You experience sukha, and then tos'a, until the desire happens to arise again in your mind.

'Ananda,' as differentiated from 'sukha,' refers to a state of spiritual bliss or joy that lies beyond the scope of relativity and the play of opposites. It is experienced when one's individual psychic flow merges with the unconditioned awareness of universal consciousness:

> Regarding Brahma (infinite, unconditioned consciousness) it has been said, "Ánandaṁ Brahma", i.e. Ánanda and Brahma are identical… a subtle line of demarcation between sukha (happiness) and ananda (bliss) has been drawn. Sukha denotes a congenial mental state whereas Ánanda is a metempirical state of bliss which overflows the mind – a state which should be called neither congenial nor uncongenial. The state of bliss is always above the scope of mind because it is limitless. The experience of bliss transcends the scope of the mind… Brahma is the name given to the ultimate quality of happiness.[3]

As one advances ever closer to this state of Ananda, it permeates one's existence in a way that is beyond the scope of happiness and sadness, sukha and dukha.

Santos'a is the internal side of aparigraha, the state of mental balance gained from understanding the use and limits of material objects and the pleasure derived from them. In the same sense as in aparigraha, it is not a negation of the material world, but rather a balanced attitude towards it, according to vaeragya and viveka as already mentioned. The practice of aparigraha is designed to create the internal state of santos'a, as it recognizes that the attempt to quench human restlessness and inner searching solely through physical pleasures is not only impossible but also counter-productive. In the very process of attempting to do so, one's desires and the need to fulfil them go on increasing ad infinitum. In the effort to release inner tensions we create addictions which reproduce the same tensions over and over and search for release in ever-increasing degrees.[4]

The effort to practice aparigraha externally, combined with the inner effort to move towards 'ananda,' the experience of which in and of itself creates a sense of inner satisfaction and gratitude for the simple things in life, works like a kind of alchemy to produce the state of santos'a. The inner-growth that this produces, instead of instant sensual-gratification and a constant search for stimulation in order to fulfil a pervasive sense of lack or avoid self-reflection and the processing of painful experiences or personal deficiencies, creates a special kind of 'happiness' which does not deny the varied expressions and emotions of life, but rather looks deeper into them to find meaning and perspective.

On a purely practical level santos'a can refer, for

example, to the effort to make the most of what comes our way in life, of what we have been given: the body we are born with, or the circumstances and challenges we are presented with. Santos'a also develops as a result of knowing that one is using one's capacity to the fullest and in a constructive way.

In Sanskrit the word for human being is 'manúsya' or 'mánava', and in Bengali 'manush', which derives from 'man,' meaning 'mind.' Mind here refers to both the heart and mind, or to the entire inner psychic and emotional world, not only the intellect.[5] The implication of this entomology is that human beings are distinguished by the fact that they are predominantly psychic beings for whom psychic or subjective experiences are more important than purely physical ones.[6] We add emotional meaning and abstract value to every expression of life: eating becomes not only an act of filling the stomach, but an act of sharing, creating social links, expressing creativity and generosity; human relationships instead of being only physical, transform into expressions of love, responsibility, sacrifice, and emotional development. As the mind increasingly takes pleasure in these subtler psychic expressions of life, with the psychic then moving towards the spiritual, a space is created for santos'a to develop. On the contrary, if all importance is laid upon the experience of physical pleasure which is necessarily momentary and limited, and which is also self-centred if not attached to higher valuse of emotional and spiritual life, the mind becomes restless and dissatisfied.

The 'contentment' of santos'a does not imply passivity in the face of social injustice, nor allowing oneself to be exploited.[7] On the contrary, it provides the inner equilibrium needed to go on struggling externally against social injustice, without loosing perspective or becoming disheartened. It is an internal state of mental balance, a special sense of fullness that arises from within.

TAPAH

Tapah refers to the spirit of sacrifice for the benefit of others and the readiness to undergo difficulties in order to reach one's goal:[1] service without desire for reward or praise, without harbouring any sort of prejudice or discrimination about who is to be served, and which involves some kind of discomfort or extra exertion on the part of the person who is offering the service. Underlying this is the understanding that such efforts lead to mental expansion:

> Tapah sádhaná is, therefore, to rise above selfishness. As a rule, practice of tapah will lead to mental dilation, and this dilation will certainly help… to a large extent, in practising Iishvara Pranidhana (meditation).[2]

The word 'sacrifice' itself comes from the Latin 'sacrificium,' made up of 'sacer' (sacred, holy) and 'facio' (to do/make).[3] Whereas in Vedic and other traditions 'sacrifice' refers to the act of ritualistic offerings into fire, 'tapah' is akin to the burning of selfishness and ego in the fire of self-less service. In the same way that ahim'sá or satya involve recognising oneself in the other, and a denial of the validity of the life and hopes of the other amounts to a denial of the same in one's self, tapah too is a recognition of the essence of divinity and desire for growth that lies in every individual, with the added implication of rising above oneself by taking on something of the suffering of the other in order to facilitate their development and consequent happiness.

Fundamentally, any kind of commitment, whether to others or to one's own principles and ideals involves some level of sacrifice. To bring up a family, to study, to do anything which is based on more than pure narcissism is, at least at the superficial level, to give up something of one's individual freedom. What is gained, however, is of immeasurable value in contrast to the loss. The freedom that is lost is an apparent and illusory one: the freedom gained that of rising above the limitations of the self, of growth through sacrifice based on the deepest meaning of love. This love is not based on personal likes and dislikes: it is universal and innate, does not discriminate and seeks no reward but rather serves as its own reward.

Anandamurti describes the importance and benefit of tapah in a very subtle and interesting way, explaining that when human activities are not guided by discernment (or viveka, as already explained in the section on satya), they are inevitably guided by instinct, like a car driven by a blind driver. The practice of tapah guided by proper discernment changes the course of human actions and sentiments.[4] A sense of love is aroused within, which is in essence a love for the divine consciousness in the one who is being served. This love is termed as 'devotion' and is the most highly prized asset on the spiritual path. Once this subtle inner feeling is gained, meditation is no longer a discipline or a distant ideal. It becomes in itself an act of love, as the mind is pulled by the force of deep inner joy towards the infinite, just as the will-force of someone in love moves unconsciously towards the thought of the beloved:

> Those who look upon the served only as the expression of the Cosmic... selflessly develop devotion or love for the Supreme in a short time. When love is aroused, and devotional sentiment is expressed, what else remains to be achieved?[5]

Readiness to undergo difficulties on the path towards a higher goal is part and parcel of discovering what it means to be truly human, and being human is to grow beyond oneself:

> ...fortunately for man the easiest path is not his truest path... man, when confronted with difficulties has to acknowledge that he is a man, that he has responsibilities to the higher faculties of his nature, by ignoring which he may achieve success that is immediate, perhaps, but that will become a death-trap to him. For what are obstacles to the lower creatures are opportunities to the higher life of man.[6]

Tapah also serves as the external and practical expression of the internal confrontation with our personal limitations and prejudices which forms a part of tantric meditation for mental expansion. The internal and external aspects of this effort are intimately interconnected and each serves as a test of the veracity of the other.[7] Tapah is an acknowledgement that struggle is a part of life and carries its own innate value. It is not something to be avoid but to be embraced, knowing all the possibilities of unfolding that it holds. Better still is to face these inner and outer struggles in the process of useful work, where they are not experienced as suffering but instead as the satisfaction of service, than to wait for them to arrive as pain without any apparent purpose.

To be productive on the practical collective level, tapah requires study and knowledge of the economic, cultural and social realities the people and locality to be served. This careful observation, planning, and sensitivity are also part of the practice of tapah. Tapah is not service only in order to make oneself 'feel good,' but service which should bring about a constructive result and be carried out even though the process yields challenges and does not flatter the ego.

The experience of one volunteer worker of the international development organization AMURT[7] can be used as an example in this respect. Dada Rudreshvarananda ('Dada' from here on) had been working in Burkina Faso in Africa since 1985. He was managing a variety of rural community-development projects in the Sahel Desert, an extremely impoverished region of the country. These projects had been built up slowly over the years through planning and consciousness raising as Dada lived and moved among the villagers. His funds were minimal, but he was always present with the people and understood the local situation well. In 1991 a large Dutch organization arrived in the region with ten million dollars to spend on 'development.' They began organizing many courses to train the villagers in modern agricultural practices, paying the villagers six dollars a day to attend the classes and eight dollars for transport. This was a huge amount of money when most had only been earning ten dollars per month. The villagers walked to the training classes, received the money and returned to their villages, generally without changing any of their agricultural practices. The presence of this organization distributing large amounts of money began to cause all kinds of corruption in the provincial population. Meanwhile, Dada, seeing that the money was doing more harm than good, went to the Dutch embassy in order to try to convince them to close the project. After four years, which was half of the planned time for the work, a review reported that eighty percent of the project had been a failure. The project director resigned, but the problems continued, as there was still five million dollars to be spent. They decided to convert one of the villages into a tourist site, and built latrines on top of what Dada described as a 'beautiful sand dune', to be used by the tourists as they rode by on camels. The tourists, not surprisingly, never arrived.

The Dutch organization also ran a literary drive, which again, caused more harm than good. Unaware of sensitive historical and cultural issues surrounding the local languages, their campaign opened up old tribal divisions which AMURT had helped to neutralize through past literacy campaigns which had united rival ethnic groups. All in all, the Dutch project was a disaster, as they had too much money to spend and wanted to show quick results without taking the time to know the local situation, and were not prepared to undertake the often slow path of patience and struggle that real change involves.[8]

Service and sacrifice in the spirit of Tapah cannot be mere tokenism, and is not done for show. It has to come from the heart, and be carried out with proper judgement, which comes from having one's own 'sweat and blood' mingled with the work. The size of the task at hand is not of importance, but the sincerity and selflessness of the sacrifice is, and this is what distinguishes it from any other kind of work.

65

SVÁDHYÁYA

Svádhyáya is the practice of study and reflection, specifically in relation to spiritual philosophy and wisdom. It is study with the intention of internalizing the inner import of what is being learnt.[1] 'Svá' literally means 'own', or 'pertaining to one's self' and 'dhyáya' 'study' or 'contemplation.' Svádhyáya is therefore 'self-study,' which implicitly also becomes 'contemplation of the self,' due to the nature of what is being studied and the style of going about it.

The importance of this point of the Niyama's can be understood first of all by considering why it forms a part of Yama-Niyama and ethics at all. In the same way that through the practice of tapah, perception and love are developed through struggle, svadhayaya produces a kind of mental friction which creates an expansion of awareness intellectually and spiritually. New ideas react with old ones, or with rigid established patterns, they clash, talk and sometimes fight with each other, and as a result one's level and depth of understanding is thus refined. In a certain sense it is the ethical responsibility of each individual to provoke this process of psychic development so that the mind does not fall into a static state and create intellectual or spiritual dogmas with their corresponding harmful social consequences. Knowledge approached in this way rests upon a base of humility and remains dynamic.

The specific reference to svádhyáya as the study of spiritual philosophy also has it reasons. From an epistemological perspective, yoga philosophy divides knowledge into various categories, and the approach to learning differs accordingly. For example, an analytical approach is coherent with the study of material sciences, but for the study of spiritual philosophy, a different and subtler kind of perception is required. The simplest division of knowledge is into 'apará' and 'pará' categories: knowledge of the external world which 'seeks to subjectivize the external objectivity' and knowledge of the self which 'aims at the subjectivization of the internal objectivity.'[2]   Apará or material knowledge is necessary and important for organization of the material world and to maintain a balance between the internal and external, the subjective inner world and the objective external one. [3] However, just as everything in the material world is relative and ever-changing, and what was reality yesterday may be obliterated tomorrow, so too apará knowledge contains innately within it the same limitations.   It can lead us to the edge of those limitations but not beyond: from there we must be at once humble and brave enough to the leap into the internal, subtle and abstract world of the self as it seeks to comprehend the nature of its own existence.

Pará knowledge, unlike apará, seeks an understanding of that which is beyond relativity: pure consciousness, unconditioned and limitless. It is an explanation, necessarily symbolic to a certain degree, sourced from the highest possible state of awareness which we have yet to obtain but aspire towards, and of all the different processes and states of experience in the process of attaining it. Spiritual philosophy, in the true sense of the term, must contain within it ever profounder levels of meaning, so that each time one deepens one's comprehension of a concept, new layers of possibility open up to be explored. This process necessarily goes hand in hand with an actual spiritual practice as part of daily life, as the two complement and give meaning to each other. Such a kind of philosophy is very different, in fact the opposite to, a dogmatic religious approach in the name of 'spirituality,' which by proclaiming unquestionable truths blocks the natural curiosity and rationality of the human mind and finishes the spiritual search before it has hardly started. The spiritual path is an endeavour in which 'the more one knows, the more one knows one does not know': breaking our own limits of perception we become aware of our ignorance and also of the untouched depths that still remain to be known, and dedicate ourselves to the continuous quest for psychic expansion. Expressed in another way:

> The transcendent is that which we bump up against when we realize our ignorance, and so it is that which transcends our ignorance... Error is the transcendent that reveals itself: what is actually revealing itself is the reality which is outside and underneath your perception.[4]

Svádhyáya builds a base upon which we can better understand and rationalize the experiences produced through spiritual practice, and meditation provides the changes in perception and experiences necessary to fully appreciate the subtleties of spiritual philosophy. In both processes, we go on 'bumping up against' the transcendent and continuously realizing our ignorance, and making efforts to overcome it. Integrating this process as part of normal life has implications not only in personal but also in collective life, and in all other areas of knowledge. When we take this attitude on the spiritual level, naturally it trickles down and permeates every other level: in the arenas of science, sociology, culture or psychology, we will remember that knowledge is acquired through a process of error, even or perhaps especially scientific knowledge, and that its value lies exactly in this recognition, in the challenging of the paradigms of current understanding considered as 'truth' so that no form of knowledge crystallises into blind and unquestioned belief. The same can be said of social movements: if we have the capacity to search for unconditioned consciousness within ourselves through challenging our own limits of perception and experience, it becomes easy to recognize the relative nature of social structures and also social struggles. We will not have to create a 'religion' out of social, political or economic movements, seeking a false security or permanence where it cannot be found. Instead we will become increasingly capable of recognizing the utility and relevance (or not) of structures and systems in the given context and discard or transform them as the context demands. In this way as a society we can surpass the tendency to reactive social movements and seek a more coherent base for social progress.

In the history of Yoga, 'philosophy' was basically always considered as an explanation of actual experiences gained through 'sádhaná', or intuitional spiritual practices. It is an attempt to explain to others certain experiences of reality and consciousness that have actually occurred. Philosophy, psychology and practice are inseparably intertwined, with the first two resulting from the wisdom gained through the latter.[5] 'Practice' here includes all aspects of spiritual meditation, which involve the systematic observation of the mind and the act of transforming one's cognitive processes, of the mind's activities and styles of perception, the interconnection between body and mind, and the interactions between the subjective and objective worlds. These observations are then systematized and expressed as philosophy. In this paradigm, 'practice' and 'theory' have never been and can never be considered as totally separate. Here in this place of meeting between philosophy, psychology and practice, there is also another meeting: of fact, meaning and experience. It is because of this meeting of the different tributaries of life that svádhyáya is not only a study of theories, but a study of the self and the meaning of the existence of that self in both subjective and objective spheres. To keep alive this study and inner search and integrate it as a part of daily life, to stimulate the growth that this produces, is considered as a basic necessity and responsibility of each individual, and for this reason it is included as a part of the ethical base of yoga with the goal of the formation of a subtle and balanced mental state.

Each age has its own aesthetic, as does each cultural context and indeed each individual. The same human search can be expressed in myriad different styles, and this should always be kept in mind as we try to penetrate the meaning of spiritual ideas and judge their validity. Throughout history the essence of yoga and tantric philosophy has been expressed equally through precise and meticulous logic and also codified in song and poetry in symbolic devotional language.[6]

There have likewise been more recent efforts to link the scientific language of physics and the abstract symbolism of mathematics with the philosophical and metaphysical language of yoga.[7] Whatever style may be used, the language will always be unavoidably symbolic as it tries to explain subtle subjective experiences and to put into words states which are in fact trans-personal and beyond the scope of individual consciousness, and therefore beyond words.

One obvious example of highly symbolic language use is the 'sandhyabhasa' or esoteric 'twilight-language' of certain tantric texts and mystical songs. 'Twilight' is of course literally the space between day and night, and symbolically, the meeting point of known and unknown, and twilight language is a codified language designed to be explained by a qualified teacher and understood by practising disciples. To give just one of many possible examples, there is a short verse in Bengali which literally translates as:

"The courtyard went into the inner room – O honourable lady, do you understand? As a result of the courtyard going inside the room, the thief that was hiding in the courtyard also went inside and stole your earrings."[8]

Underlying the superficial meaning, which appears nonsensical, the verse is actually explaining the process of introversion of the dispersed, extroverted mind. As a result of spiritual sádhaná, the outer world (the courtyard) or superficial aspects of the mind are focused internally and merged with the inner subconscious and then unconscious layers of the mind, and the individual then merges into the universal (the inner room). As a result, all limitations of perception, mental complexes and suffering disappear ('are stolen away') in this state of perfect fullness. It can also be added that the 'thief' (cosmic consciousness personified) had been hiding all along even in the external world, (the courtyard) but due to the dispersion of the mind was not perceived.[9]

Of course, not all explanations of spiritual philosophy use such colourful and cryptic language, but such an example makes it easy to understand how ideas can be misunderstood if not internalized and contemplated deeply upon. Zen koans, or Sufi and Baul songs, are other examples of cryptic or poetic language used to express the inexpressible. Even when a more general format is used, the same process of reflection to understand the essence of the words is necessary, as whatever manages to be expressed inevitably contains many layers of meaning and even then is only a small part of the actual experience attempted to be relayed.

IISHVARA PRAN'IDHÁNA

Iishvara pran'idhána, the final point of Yama-Niyama, is both the base and source of inspiration for all the previous nine points, as well as their goal. 'Iishvara' is Cosmic Consciousness, pure and unconditioned, both transcendent and also immanent, the experience of which is perfect fullness, the bliss and ultimate freedom of completeness without lack. Iishvara is both the witnessing consciousness and the essence of all that exists: hidden in the superficialities of the ever-changing material and external world, and revealed within the deepest essence of the introverted self. [1] 'Pran'idhána' means 'to understand clearly or to adopt something as a shelter.'[2] Therefore 'Iishvara pran'idhána' literally means 'to accept Iishvara, Cosmic Consciousness, as one's shelter' or to 'gain a clear understanding' of 'Iishvara,' with the implication that this understanding comes from knowing intimately or merging oneself with that which one is trying to understand. Practically, it is the effort to identify one's individual mental flow with infinite consciousness and unify one's sense of existence with that flow.[3] This is both the process and goal of spiritual meditation or 'sádhaná.' It is a concept as well as an actual technique, and the effort which all other yogic practices are a preparation for: it is the actual meaning of 'yoga' as 'union.'[4]

Everything that we generally identify with so strongly as human beings is transitory: our physical possessions, relationships, physical body, psychic qualities and thought patterns. Our cultural, social and gender identities are also only fluctuating and restricted versions of 'who we are.' This is not to say that they are insignificant, but that they are not nearly as significant as we think they are, and certainly are not permanent. They are important and necessary in and as far as we understand their limitations. Understanding this, they can be guided to serve a higher purpose, but taken as the core of our identity become a source of insecurity, conflict or attachment and obscure our clarity of vision.   What we hold on to today as the centre of our personal identity may change drastically with time. The stronger we cling to such identities, the more enforced and difficult to change they become, and when due to some or other alteration of circumstances these walls of dependency on which our 'self' is leaning fall away, the greater will be the shock as one is forced to reassess everything they so staunchly believed they innately were. Life itself, be it desired it or not, forces this reassessment upon us, sometimes softly and patiently, other times suddenly and with harsh blows.

If, in the depths of the self, we realize that fundamentally we are something more that our transitory identity, that we are created from and ensconced in some other intangible and infinite mystery, and succeed step by step in identifying with this essence, then internally we become both unbreakable even in the most difficult of circumstances and also mentally free. Even if all the walls upon which one leans upon as a person acting in the relative world are removed, still one will remain standing, as one's final support is an internal centre, holding the personality together just as the spine holds up the physical frame.

Such an abstract concept as 'Cosmic Consciousness' naturally begins as little more than an idea, perhaps felt intuitively or deduced through a process of logic.   This sprout of an idea needs to be stabilized and its veracity established through the inner experience of each individual. A personal connection must be established with the said flow of consciousness, and in doing so, the individual will discover something so deep and beautiful that they will not fear to loose any smaller things of life, those things of temporary value, in order to hold on to that experience. If this inspiration is the base of one's morality, then one's ethical ideals will become internalized and will hold together even in moments of adversity. A person becomes fearless, self-inspired, and begins to live in the fullness of being.

Spiritual meditation is the systematic training of the mind towards such a heightened state of consciousness, not only spontaneously, but as a normal part of daily life. It involves a particular method through which the mind is detached first of all from the external world, the physical body and the superficial thought patterns of the mind. The dispersed mind is collected together, and then the 'I-feeling', the totality of one's sense of self-identity, is focused at a point. From this point one's identity is guided to flow with and is transformed into Cosmic Consciousness. This is done through the use of mantra, a set of specially chosen sound-vibrations connected to a conceptual idea, which guides the mind toward ever deeper layers of the self:

'...this feeling of 'I am' having been developed and

expressed spontaneously is then transformed into the feeling of Brahma (infinite consciousness). This spontaneous idea is not easily understood by those who do not practise sádhaná (spiritual meditation).[5]

This is a subtle endeavour, brought about through the internal channelization of feelings in a directed yet also natural and spontaneous way that will be experienced uniquely by each individual. The actual techniques are taught in a personalized process of initiation, which involves a mental re-orientation on the part of the student, who at the moment of learning accepts the spiritual path and discipline as an integral part of human life.[6] There are also introductory techniques which help to lead-up to this point.[7]

Human creative energy, if it does not have an outlet or a purpose, conspires to create a kind of internal friction which seeks all manners and styles of release. It seeks fleeting excitement, many times self-destructive in excess, or countless novel ways to 'forget' the existential tensions and dilemmas of being, desiring a kind of negative freedom or momentary oblivion. In this case, the potential and creativity of the human mind is released, but without producing anything of lasting value, internally or externally. Iishvara pran'idhána collects this creative force and guides it inwardly, opening up the potential of the mind in ever-increasing degrees. This process, aside from its ultimate spiritual goal, naturally induces many secondary benefits along the way, transforming the emotional and thus neurological processes as all the tendencies of the human mind gradually find their harmonious place within the whole. Thus our creative energy, instead of being discharged and lost, has the chance to fulfil itself as the catalyst for a transformation of the inner subjective state. This change can then be expressed as practical and constructive acts of ingenuity and conscientiousness in the external world. This internal change creates a unique blissful or pleasurable experience which is different from the normal transient or external-materially oriented understanding of 'pleasure.' It is special in that one experiences pleasure through the process of increased self awareness, becoming 'more aware of thoughts and feelings conceptually, but less emotionally disrupted by them.'[8] Possessing the tools to guide the mind and grow inwardly, one need no longer fear ones inner processes nor seek to avoid them. The deep satisfaction thus gained from being capable of using the mind to surpass itself produces a new kind of security, freedom, and joy: happiness in the real sense of the word, of a variety that is resilient even amidst sadness, struggle or pain.

There are an almost endless variety of different ways in which the meaning and process of Iishvara pran'idhána could be described: in psychological language describing the cognitive and perceptive changes it involves; in metaphysical or philosophical terminology; or in the mystical-devotional language as a journey of rapture, love and union with the universal soul. All of these are equally valid. Perhaps the best explanation, and in the least words, would be simply to say that at the heart of creation lies a great mystery, human life is a journey to penetrate the essence of that mystery, and Iishvara pran'idhána is the conscious acceptance of this intangible truth and journey.

The human mind needs a foundation upon which to

base its movement, thoughts and decisions. This foundation serves as a mirror upon which we can observe ourselves, and also as a catalyst to self-reflection and growth. Yet what base is there which will not at some point limit us, which does not risk falling into rigidity and dogma? The word 'ideology' in general has negative connotations, implying a fixed world-view which clouds the analytical abilities, imposing preconceived conclusions upon reality. Upon what then shall we structure our thinking and values? To reject any kind foundation for our mental or subjective orientation is also a kind of dogma which carries with it its own danger, as new, unconscious beliefs are unavoidably created even as we deny possessing them. Perhaps, just perhaps, there is one base upon which we can fearlessly build: upon the idea of life as a process of continuous mental expansion, challenging our own limitations as we attempt to penetrate ever deeper into the mystery of creation and the self. If our ideas flow forth from this process they remain dynamic and vital, ever refining themselves, inspired from the tangential point between known and unknown, finite and infinite.

Anandamurti, in defining the word 'ideology' proposed exactly this: a redefinition of the concept itself, based on the Sanskrit word 'adarsha.' He proposed ideology as being the conceptualization of the 'bháva', or 'ideational flow', through which the vibrations of the individual mind are straightened to merge into the infinite. The experience and inspiration of that 'bháva', that infinite, unrestricted and unconditioned flow of consciousness, translated into thought and idea, becomes 'ideology'.[9] Ideology then, in this spiritual-yogic sense, is having as our mental base that flow of thought which ever expands the mind beyond its limited conditioning until it merges into unconditioned consciousness. Or restated in more pragmatic terms: the base of life as a process of internal self-realization expressed externally through service to the entire created world. In this way, we take as our orientation that which continuously throws off our limitations, misconceptions and preconceptions.

Thus we return to where we started: the inspiration of Iishvara pran'idhána, defined as the act of embracing the journey towards comprehending the mystery of life, functions as the subtle source of inspiration for all of Yama-Niyama; and Yama-Niyama as the ethical foundation for mental equilibrium, the expansion of empathy and love, and for a civilization and culture which creates the space in which human capacity and potential can fully express themselves. This process of expansion of love goes on refining our ethics, just as simultaneously our ethical principles refine our experience and understanding of love, and in this way we proceed to the highest pinnacle of the self, and become human beings filled with joy.

<u>NOTES</u>

<u>Introduction</u>

1. 'So on your plane of morality, there are two divisions: psycho-physical emanation and physico-psychic movement. In Sanskrit, this psycho-physical emanation is called Yama and physico-psychic movement is called Niyama.' (Anandamurti, 'The Cult of Spirituality', Subhasita Samgraha Part 18)

2. For example, the 'Sandilya Upanishad' lists ten Yamas, the first five of which are identical to those in the Patainjali Sutras. At least 65 ancient texts are known that discuss the Yamas and Niyamas. (See SV Bharti, 2001, Pg. 680.691)

3. Ananda Marga is a socio-spiritual organization founded in 1955 by Shrii Shrii Anandamurti, combining the goals of 'self-realization and service to humanity', for a spirituality based on practice and rationality and a society which promotes the integrated physical, mental and spiritual development of the individual and collective.   The fundamental philosophical ideas of Ananda Marga can be found in the books 'Ananda Sutram' and 'Ananda Marga Elementary Philosophy.'

4. 'In Western philosophy observance of ethical principles is considered the primary goal in life, but Ananda Marga philosophy considers that ethical observance is the primary step towards the higher life. Niiti or principle is not the goal of human life, rather it is a starting point of life's journey.' (Anandamurti, 'Tattva Kaomudii Part 2')

5. Neohumanism is a world-view characterized by love for the Supreme. In the early stages of developing one's spiritual devotion, the adoption of Neohumanistic principles – that is, abjuring all prejudices against other races, groups, religions, and less-evolved creatures – will safeguard and enhance the development of that devotion.

And once, in turn, a person comes to feel devotion for the Supreme, that devotion or love will ultimately overflow onto all objects created by the Supreme. One will come spontaneously to love all beings and objects as one loves the Supreme, free from any discrimination.

So devotion expands one's world-view, and the more expansive the world-view, the more one finds the ecstasy and peace of devotion.' (Sarkar, 'Neohumanism, Liberation of Intellect.')

6. Towsey, 2011, Pg. 41

7. Towsey, 2011, Pg. 41

8. 'Morality is the foundation of Sádhaná (spiritual practice). It must, however, be remembered that morality or good conduct is not the culminating point of the spiritual march. As a moralist one may set an ideal for other moralists, but to do this is not something worth mentioning for a Sádhaka (spiritual aspirant). Sádhaná, in its very start, requires mental equilibrium. This sort of mental harmony may also be termed as morality.' (Anandamurti, 'A Guide to Human Conduct.')

9. 'Morality depends on one's efforts to maintain a balance regarding time, place and person, and therefore there may be differences in the moral code.' (Anandamurti, 'A Guide to Human Conduct.')

10. Rudolf, 2017, Loc 892.

11. Anandamurti, 'Ananda Sutram', sutra 2-14.

12. '...the individual should feel a fraternal emotion for and attachment to the external world. This sentimental contact with the external world is a must. If someone is under the impression that "I am doing sádhaná for the sake of personal liberation and I have nothing to do with the world," and thus denies his or her contact with external physicality, although the person's physical body is very much in this world, the person is cheating himself and indulging in selfishness. Service to humanity with a view to serve Parama Puruśa and with the same attachment which one feels towards oneself and Parama Puruśa is an essential prerequisite for progress in sádhaná. This will establish the equilibrium and parallelism

of the individual rhythms with the rhythms of the external physicalities.' (Anandamurti, 'Mantra Caetanya,' Subhasita Samgraha Part 10)

13.   'Sutra 3-10. Vádhá sá yuśamáná shaktih sevyaṁ sthápayati lakśye. [Obstacles are the helping forces that establish one in the goal.]

Purport: Obstacles in fact are no foes on the path of sádhaná [spiritual practice], but indeed friends. They only do service to a person. It is on account of these obstacles that the battle rages against them, and this counter-effort alone carries the sádhaka [spiritual aspirant] to his or her cherished goal.' (Anandamurti, 'Ananda Sutram')

14.   'Tantra finds or creates circumstances designed expressedly to bring out, rather than to intern away, one's problematic mental tendencies.' (Anandamurti, 'Discourses on Tantra Part 1')

15. Anandamurti, 'Guide to Human Conduct.'

16. Towsey, 2011, Pg. 41

17. 'Sutra 2-5. Tasminnupalabdhe paramá trśńánivrttih.
[That (Brahma) having been attained, all thirst is permanently quenched.]

Purport: There is in the living being a thirst for limitlessness. It is not possible for limited objects to quench one's thirst. Brahma is the only limitless entity, and so establishment in Brahma's bearing alone puts an end to all thirsts or cravings.' (Anandamurti, 'Ananda Sutram.')

18. See, for example, Zamyatin, 'We', 1924.

19. See, for example, Lem, 'The Futurological Congress', 1974 and Huxley, 'Brave New World', 2002.

20. Anandamurti proposes that human progress takes place through 'Physical clash, psychic clash, and attraction to the Great.' The first two are forced upon us by pressure of circumstances, and the third takes place through the propulsion of our own positive desire.

'I said that for microcosmic progress three factors are indispensable – physical clash, psychic clash and attraction of the Great.

Whenever there is clash or conflict within any structure, whether subtle or crude, it acquires subtlety. This applies to both psychic clash and physical clash. The more subtle the crude mind becomes as a result of internal clash, the greater its spiritual awakening.' (Anandamurti, 'Subhasita Samgraha 7', discourse: 'Cosmic Attraction and Spiritual Cult.')
21. Maturana, 2008, Pg. 221
22. Maturana, 2008, Pg. 138
23. Maturana, 2008, Pg. 223

<u>AHIMSA</u>
1. Anandamurti, 'A Guide to Human Conduct.'
2. '*Manovákkáyaeh sarvabhútá námapiidá namahim'sá*'- (Anandamurti, 'A Guide to Human Conduct.') 'Sarva' means all and 'bhútá' refers to the created world, hence 'all of creation.'
3. 'According to this interpretation, ahim'sá means non-application of force. Possibly it is this interpretation which has distorted most the meaning of ahim'sá. In all actions of life, whether small or big, the unit mind progresses by surmounting the opposing forces. Life evolves through the medium of force.' (Anandamurti, 'A Guide to Human Conduct')
4. 'When there is any application of force, it cannot be called non-violence. Is it not violence if you hurt a person not by your own hands but by some other indirect means? Is the boycott movement against a particular nation not violence?' (Anandamurti, 'A Guide to Human Conduct.)
5. 'Some so-called learned persons define the word ahim'sá in such a manner that if one adheres to it strictly it becomes impossible to live not only in society but also in forests, hills or caves.' (Anandamurti, 'A Guide to Human Conduct.')
6. Tagore, 1918, 'Nationalism.'
7. 'Karma' here is a philosophically incorrect term, and has been used here in the common, albeit incorrect,

understanding of the word for the sake of understanding. 'Karma' actually mean 'action', and 'samskara' is the proper term for the reactions of ones actions.

8. Tagore, 1918, 'Nationalism.' (LOC 694)

9. Tagore, 1916, 'Sadhana.'

10. Quoted from 'Jordan Peterson vs Susan Blackmore: Do we Need God to Make Sense of Life?' https://www.youtube.com/watch?v=syP-OtdCIho

11. See Dostoyevsky, 1866, 'Crime and Punishment.'

12. 'The Shaiva method is one of ever widening inclusion of phenomena mistakenly thought to be outside the absolute. The Vedantin, on the other hand, seeks to understand the nature of the absolute by excluding (nisedha) everything which does not conform to the criterion of absoluteness, until all that remains is the unqualified Brahma. The Saiva's approach is one of affirmation and the Vedantin's one of negation.' (Dyczkowski, 1989, 'The Doctrine of Vibration.')

13. For explanations about the conscious, subconscious and unconscious mind, see the chapter and notes of 'Satya.'

14. In the yogic system, and also in Ayurvedic medicine, food is divided into three catagories depending on their effects on perception and the emotional state. These are 'sattvic' (sentient), 'rajasik' (mutative), and 'tamasik' (static). Sattvic foods promote an expansion of consciousness and subtle perception, rajasik indicates movement and change, and tamasik dullness, lack of focus, and limited perceptive capacity. Sentient food include most vegetarian foods and dairy products. Rajasik foods include items such a tea, coffee and chocolate. Tamasik food include meat, fish, eggs, onion, garlic, mushrooms and alcohol. (Note that rajasik and tamasik foods may or may not be healthy for the body, but they are considered definitely unhleathy for the mind). Yogic practice recommend a sattvik diet, with small quantities of rajasik foods if desired. For more information see: Anandamurti, 'Yoga Psychology,' chapter: 'Food, Cells and Mental Development.'

<u>SATYA</u>

1. 'Satya implies proper action of mind and right use of words with the spirit of welfare.' (Anandamurti, 'A Guide to Human Conduct.'

2. 'In the opinion of the yogic scriptures there is an ideological difference between rta and satya. That which is a fact, which has happened or happens, is called rta. And the ideation used for the welfare of the people is called satya. ' (Sarkar, 'Shabda Cayanika Part 2,' chapter 'Rka to Rksá'.)

3. Anandamurti, 'Namah Shivaya Shantaya', chapter 'The Teaching of Shiva- Part 1.'

4. 'Humans are rational beings: they possess in varying degrees the capability to do what is necessary or good for humanity. In the realm of spirituality, such thought, word or action has been defined as satya.' (Anandamurti, 'A Guide to Human Conduct.')

5. For examples of the yogic theory of mind, see: Towsey's 'Eternal Dance of Macrocosm,' (2011), or Sarkar's 'Idea and Ideology.'

6. See Towsey, 2011, Pg. 75-78; and Sarkar, 'Idea and Ideology', chapter 'Kos'a'.

7. -'This loka in the human mind is called the kámamaya kośa or the crude mind, which controls all the actions of the body. This sphere is therefore limited to all the actions connected with the body.' (Anandamurti, 'Subhasita Samgraha Part 1,' chapter 'The Call of the Supreme.')
-'In Sanskrit those physical entities with which, we say, human existence is closely coordinated is called "Káma". You cannot do without these things – food, clothing, education, medical treatment. These things are essential for human life. They come within the grasp of Káma, the lowest layer. ' (Anandamurti, 'Ananda Vacanamrtam Part 14', chapter 'Pinnacled Existence.')

8. 'The manomaya kośa is subtler than the kámamaya kośa and it has the capacity of recollection and contemplation

(smaraṅa and manana).' (Sarkar, 'Idea and Ideology', chapter 'Kos'a'.)

9. See Towsey, 2011, Pg. 77

10. This description has been taken from handwritten notes of the words of the explanations of Anandamurti to the acaryas of Ananda Marga.

11. Towsey, 2011, Pg. 76

12. Towsey, 2011, Pg. 77-78

13. Tagore, 1916, LOC 214.

14. In this context, Shippey describes Saruman as the: "most contemporary figure in Middle-earth" (see Shippey, 2002, Pg. 68-77).

15. Tolkien, 2000, Pg. 276-277

16. 'Tolkien is very careful to differentiate the rhetorical choices of the characters in The Lord of the Rings [LotR], so that, particularly in the case of Gandalf and Saruman, rhetoric is character. ' (Rudd, J, 'The Voice of Saruman.')

17. 'For progress in the spiritual realm, one must not ignore the psychic realm or the mundane external sphere. One will move steadily in the spiritual sphere, and the rjutá [straightforwardness], sáhas [courage] and satyaniśthá [love of truth] that grow as one progresses in the spiritual sphere will be utilized for the mental welfare of the entire world.' (Anandamurti, 'Subhasita Samgraha Part 24,' chapter 'Incantation and Human Progress.')

18. 'The practical side of satya is dependent on relativity, but its finality lies in Parama Brahma. That is why Brahma is often referred to as the 'essence of satya.' (Anandamurti, 'A Guide to Human Conduct.')

ASTEYA

1. 'Not to take possession of what belongs to others is asteya. It means non-stealing.' Anandamurti, 'A Guide to Human Conduct.'

2. See Anandamurti, 'A Guide to Human Conduct,' chapter 'Asteya.'

3. See Anandamurti, 'Ananda Sutram', Chapter 5; and Sarkar, 'Prout in a Nutshell' series.

4. Sarkar (Anandamurti) criticized both the capitalist system of private ownership and the communism system of communes, which he describes as being against basic human psychology. Both are purely materialistic in their world-view, and not considered conducive to subtler human and cultural development. In their place he proposed a decentralized cooperative based model which recognizes diversity and individual merit. These ideas have been outlined in series of books titled 'Prout in a Nutshell.'

BRAHMACARYA

1. Dyczkowski, 1986, 'The Doctrine of Vibration.'

2. Dyczkowski, 1986, 'The Doctrine of Vibration.'

3. See Singh,   2006, 'Vijñánabhairava or Divine Consciousness.'

-'On the occasion of such great delight or intensive experience, one should lay hold of the source of the experience, viz, the spanda or the pure spiritual throb and meditate on it till his mind is deeply steeped in it. He will then become identified with the spiritual principle.' (Verse 71, pg. 68)

-'...the emphasis is on the meditation of the source of joy which is spiritual. Leaving aside the various sensuous media, the aspirant should meditate on that fountain of all joy which only trickles in drops in all the joys of life.' (Verse 73, Pg. 69)

4. 'The beginning, the middle and end of dharma sádhaná is to rush towards Him, to channelize all the positive and negative propensities of mind toward Him. Spiritual aspirants will not destroy the six ripus (not even káma or physical longing) but will utilize them for their benefit. When utilized as aids for spiritual progress they will do no further harm. So-called jiṋánis may fight the propensity of krodha (anger), but devotees will utilize it to fight staticity.

They will shatter the meanness and pettiness of the mind through psychic strength and fearsome temper… In this way spiritual aspirants keep their vision fixed on Brahma.' (Anandamurti, 'Subhasita Samgraha Part 7, chapter 'The Macrocosmic Stance and Human Life.')

5. For example:

-The 'Sandilya Upanishad' (chapter 1) defines Brahmacarya as: 'refraining from sexual intercourse in all places and in all states of mind, speech or body.'

-Popular translations of the 'Yoga Sutras of Patainjali' also use the definiton:

'***Brahmacharya pratishtayam viaryalabhaha"*** *(II Sutra 38)*

Brahmacharya= celibacy; **Pratishtayam**= established; **Viarya** = vigour; **Iabhaha** = gained.

"On being established in celibacy vigour is gained."

('The Art of Living,' https://www.artofliving.org/uy-es/yoga/patanjali-yogasutra/knowledge-sheet-70)

6.   'In the olden times only the actual meaning of Brahmacarya was accepted.   Later, when society was dominated by the intelligentsia, the so-called monks, who had taken to complete exploitation, thought that if ordinary citizens were allowed to pursue spiritual practices, they might lose the machinery of exploitation at any moment, of which they were so fond. If common people are inspired by spiritual ideals their rationality will grow and grow.   The monks realized therefore that the people will have to be kept maimed and helpless.   Fear and inferiority complex will have to be infused in people to exploit them.   They found that such an exploited mass consisted of ordinary worldly people, most of whom were married. If, therefore, the loss of semen was anyhow declared anti-religious, they would be able to gain their end without difficulty… Ordinary worldly people began to think that they, by leading a married life, had committed a serious wrong, a heinous sin: they has indulged in activities against brahmacarya.' (Anandamurti, 'A Guide to Human Conduct.')

7. Anandamurti, 'A Guide to Human Conduct.'

8. Shrii Shrii Anandamurti, the founder of the socio-spiritual organization created a systems of 'acaryas' or celibate teachers who have dedicated their lives to social service and teaching spiritual practices and philosophy. The system involves certain lifestyle regulations, regarding food, yoga practices, mental attitudes etc. which support this practice physically and psychologically. The central purpose of the practice is the freedom and flexibility which facilitates dedication to one's ideal and to society at large. The same can be used as guidelines for those who are not acaryas but for some other reason decide to lead a single life.

9. In the social and spiritual system of Ananda Marga, marriage and family life is considered as highly respectable and beneficial to spiritual progress. Within this system, sexual relations are recommended not more than four times per month, as the ideal to create a balance between the physical, mental and spiritual aspects of life. Yogic guidelines regarding food, asanas (yoga postures), etc are also recommended to help incorporate the sexual impulses into the personality in a balanced way.

Acarya and family life are just different approaches, depending on the disposition of the person. The purpose of yogic practices relating to food, fasting, etc, is that the mind should remain focused and calm according to the lifestyle chosen, and not the development of any special power, etc.

10. In reference to the first lesson of Ananda Marga meditation, which uses the ideation that 'I am Brahma', and the second lesson, which is a technique for the conscious practice of Brahmacarya, using the ideation that 'everything is an expression of Brahma.'

11. Tagore, 1916, LOC 732.

12. Tagore 1916, LOC 782.

13. Sepehri, 2013, Pg. 59 (Poem: 'We are the Shady Bower of our Tranquillity.')

14. '...you cannot effectively indulge in the suppression or

repression of a certain Bháva for long, ultimately it overpowers you, because the more you try to suppress it the greater becomes the force with which it rebounds. If crude ideas come into your mind, you are not crude or bad – it is natural for them to come. But mental or psychic suppression or repression of these is not profitable for Sádhakas. Instead the correct and psychological approach to Máyá is to channelize it in the direction of the Absolute... Relatively speaking, absence of pain or pleasure – which is called Nirapekśavedaniiyam – is in effect psychic suppression or repression. This is an unnatural state of mind and whether it lasts five minutes or ten minutes, five days or ten days or even a period of years, when the control is removed it again bursts forth in the form of Anukulavedaniiyam or Pratikulavedaniiyam. Psychic suppression or repression, therefore, does not lead to progress.' (Sarkar, 'A Few Problems Solves Part 6', chapter: 'The Human Search for Real Progress.')

And similarly: 'When the doer "I" of the aspirant is goaded towards the Supreme Entity, it uses the vital energy... passing through different planes of inferences, and through different propensities of the human mind, without suppressing those propensities of the mind. The question of suppression, repression and oppression does not arise in the realm of spiritual cult. You are simply to maintain equilibrium and equipoise – that is, you are to move maintaining proper parallelism with the fundamental propensities of the human mind. (Anandamurti, 'Subhasita Samgraha Part 18,' chapter: 'Cult, Inference and Propensity.')

<u>APARIGRAHA</u>
1. 'Non-indulgence in the enjoyment of such amenities and comforts as are superfluous for the preservation of life is aparigraha.' (Anandamurti, 'A Guide to Human Conduct.')
2. Tagore, 1916, LOC 717.
3. Tagore, 1916, LOC 717.

4. Tagore, 1916, LOC 1274.
5. 'Vaerágya is commonly understood to mean retiring from the world and leading a life of strict self-denial by practising excessive austerity. Vaerágya does not mean this. It does not make one a recluse. It only means to attempt to understand the proper use of things and to use them correctly (of course without working under the control of the crude objects of mind only).' (Anandamurti, 'Ananda Marga: Elementary Philosophy', chapter: 'How Should Human Beings Live in this World.')
6. Anandamurti, 'Ananda Marga: Elementary Philosophy', chapter: 'How Should Human Being Live in this World.'
7. Anandamurti, 'Ananda Marga: Elementary Philosophy', chapter: 'How Should Human Being Live in this World.'
8.   Sarkar, 'Proutist Economics', chapter: 'Quadri-Dimensional Economy.'
9. PROUT (Progressive Utilization Theory), as proposed by P.R. Sarkar, is an example of one such proposed approach. Details can be found the books 'Proutist Economics' (Sarkar) and chapter 5 or 'Ananda Sutram' (Anandamurti), among others.

SHAOCA

1. 'The first aspect of Niyama Sádhaná is Shaoca. It means purity or cleanliness. It can be subdivided into two parts, one relating to the external sphere, ie., external cleanliness, and the other to the mental sphere, ie., internal cleanliness. ' (Anandamurti, 'A Guide to Human Conduct.')
2. Although this concept is popularly known as 'karma,' the correct philosophical term is 'samskara.' 'Karma' literally mean 'action', whereas 'samskara' is 'reaction is potentiality.'
   'Manovikrtih vipákápekśitá saṁskárah.
[A distortion of the mind-stuff waiting for expression (i.e., a reaction in potentiality) is known as a saṁskára.]' (Anandamurti, 'Ananda Sutram,' chapter 3, sutra 4.)
3. 'Virtuous or non-virtuous, whatever the act may be, it

begets a sort of mental distortion. The mind, however, regains its normal composure through vipáka, after undergoing the consequences of one's good or bad deeds. Where action has taken place, but the consequences thereof have not been gone through or served, that is, the vipáka has been kept in abeyance, such suspended or deferred vipáka is called saṁskára [reaction in its potentiality].' (Anandamurti, 'Ananda Sutram', chapter 3, sutra 4.)

4. 'When people, driven by instincts, direct their mental stuff blindly towards the objects of pleasure without taking help from their conscience- or when mind ultimately gets crudified by being constantly goaded by selfish motives- whether or not they think of doing harm to others, their mind gets distorted. The complexes by which this distortion occurs are the dirts of the mind.' (Anandamurti, 'A Guide to Human Conduct.')

5. 'The relation between the physical body and the mind is very close. Mental expression is brought about through the vrttis, and the predominance of the vrttis depends on different glands of the body. There are many glands in the body and from each there is a secretion of a particular hormone. If there is any defect in the secretion of hormones or any defect in a gland, certain vrttis become excited. For this reason, we find that in spite of having a sincere desire to follow the moral code, many persons cannot do so; they understand that they should do meditation, but they cannot concentrate their minds because their minds become extroverted due to the external excitement of this or that propensity. If a person wants to control the excitement of these propensities, he or she must rectify the defects of the glands. Ásanas help the sádhaka to a large extent in this task, so ásanas are an important part of sádhaná.' (Anandamurti, 'Ananda Marga Caryacarya Part 3', chapter 'Asanas')

6. See, for example, 'the 16 points' as given in the book 'Caryacarya Part 2,' (Anandamurti).

7. For a list of the 'vrttis' or tendencies associated with each

cakra, see: Anandamurti, 'Yoga Psychology', discourse: 'Plexi and Microvita.')

8. As explained in the notes on Ahim'sá.

9. See Huxley, 2002, 'A Brave New World.'

10. Anandamurti, 'Subhasita Samgraha Part 10', chapter 'Taking the Opposite Stance in Battle.'

11. Anandamurti, 'Caryacarya Part 2.'

<u>SANTOS'A</u>

1. 'Tos'a means a state of mental ease. Santos'a, therefore, means a state of proper ease.' (Anandamurti, 'A Guide to Human Conduct.')

2. -See Anandamurti, 'Ananda Sutram', Chapter 2, Sutra 1: '*Anukúlavedaniiyaḿ sukham.* [A congenial mental feeling is called happiness.] Purport: If the mental waves of someone whose saḿskára happens to be the quiescent form of those waves, find similar waves emanating either from any crude object or from any other mind-entity, then those waves, in that person's case, are said to be complementary and reciprocal. The contact of these mutually-sympathetic waves is what is called happiness.'

-And sutras 3 and 4: *'Sukhamanantamánandam.* [Infinite happiness is ánanda (bliss).] Purport: No living being is content with a little, not to speak of human beings. And so, small happiness fills nobody's bill. One wants endless happiness. This endless happiness is a condition beyond the precincts of weal and woe, because the sense of happiness that is perceivable with the help of the senses oversteps the limit of the sense organs when established in limitlessness. This limitless happiness is what is known as ánanda [bliss].

Ánandaḿ Brahma ityáhuh. [This ánanda is called Brahma.]'

-See also Anandamurti, 'Subhasita Samgraha 24', discourse 'Bhakti, Mukti and Parama Purusa': 'When one comes in contact with another object and after coming in contact with that object a sympathetic psychic vibration is created, and that sympathetic psychic vibration maintains a parallelism with the physical vibration of that object, then we say it is sukham [pleasure, happiness]. And when the psychic vibration of a person cannot maintain parallelism with the physical vibration of that object, then we say it is duhkham [pain, sorrow]... And when the wavelength of sukha, the wavelength of the sympathetic vibration, becomes almost infinite, that is, becomes straightened just like a straight line, then it is sukham anantam [endless happiness]. It is ánandam.'

3. Anandamurti, 'Tattva Kaomudii Part 2.'

4. 'As a result of extroversial analysis, the objects of enjoyment go on increasing both in number and abstraction and that's why one's mental flow never gets any rest. Under such circumstances, how can one attain perfect peace of mind?' (Anandamurti, 'A Guide to Human Conduct.')

5. -'*Mon*, from the Sanskrit *Manas*; in colloquial Bengali it implies both heart and mind; to the Bául it represents himself, symbolizing heart and mind, spirit and matter.' (Bhattacarya, D. 1999)

-'In human beings the jiivátmá is far more developed that in any other creature, because the mind is far more developed than in any other creature. That is why human beings are called "manúsya" or "mánava". "Mana" + "u" + "sna" = "mánava", the entity where mind dominates, and not matter.' (Anandamurti, 'Ananda Vacanamrtam 3,' discourse 'Sadgurum Tam Namami.')

6. 'Human beings are called mánuśya or mánuśa, etc. They are called by terms in which the word mana [mind] occurs in one form or other, because the human is a mana-pradhána [mind-dominated] creature. They are beings in whom the mind and thinking are the predominant moving forces, and in whom the instinct does not play the role which it plays in the other animals.' (Anandamurti, 'Ananda Vacanamrtam 7', discourse 'The Mana-Pradhana Creature.')

7. 'Santos'a Sádhaná does not imply that you should allow yourself to be exploited or oppressed by someone who takes advantage of your simplicity, and you should tolerate it silently. It is by no means proper for you to give up your right to self-preservation or your legitimate dues in life. You have to go on fighting with concerted efforts for the establishment of your rights. But you must never violate the principle of santos'a by wasting your physical and mental energy under the sway of excessive greed.' (Anandamurti, 'A Guide to Human Conduct.')

TAPAH
1. 'Tapah means efforts to reach the goal despite such efforts being associated with physical discomforts.' (Anandamurti, 'Idea and ideology,' chapter 'The place of sadvipras in the samaja cakra.')
2. Anandamurti, 'A Guide to Human Conduct.'
3. https://en.wiktionary.org/wiki/sacrifice
4. 'There is another peculiarity in tapah. When the activities of human beings are not guided by discrimination, they are goaded by instinct. Tapah guided by discrimination changes the course of action and leads people towards emancipation. Of course, devotion also gives rise to discrimination but such devotion cannot be aroused in those who have not experienced Cosmic bliss.' (Anandamurti, 'A Guide to Human Conduct.')
5. Anandamurti, 'A Guide to Human Conduct.'
6. Tagore, 1918, LOC 39.
7.   -'It is not only an external or internal fight, it is simultaneously both. The internal fight is a practice of the subtler portion of Tantra. The external fight is a fight of the cruder portion of Tantra. And the fight both external and internal is a fight in both ways at once. So practice in each and every stratum of life receives due recognition in Tantra. ... The practice for raising the kulakuńdalinii is the internal sádhaná of Tantra, while shattering the bondages of hatred,

suspicion, fear, shyness, etc., by direct action is the external sádhaná.' (Anandamurti, 'Discourses on Tantra Volume 2', chapter: 'Tantra and its Effect on Society.')

-'...all Tantrics are brought face to face with their weaknesses in one way or other. A Tantric guru assigns to his disciples tremendous responsibilities for social change. The disciples' participation in an activist movement aimed at a just and spiritually-based society forces them to confront sometimes physical fear, but more routinely the fear of social censure and the fear of the overwhelming task before them. The inferiority complex is the most debilitating fear which most of us must learn to overcome in our lives.' (Anandamurti, 'Discourses on Tantra Volume 2,' 'Publisher's Note.')

8. For the complete account of events relating to this example, see:

www.anandamarga.net/archive/rudreshvarananda.htm

<u>SVÁDHYÁYA</u>

1. 'Svadhayaya means not only to read or hear a subject, but to understand its significance, the underlying idea.' (Anandamurti, 'A Guide to Human Conduct.')

2. (Anandamurti, 'Ananda Vacanamrtam 33' discourse: 'Pará and Apará Knowledge.')

3. What Anandamurti defined as 'subective approach and objective adjustment,' necessary for balance for balance in spiritual and practical life. (See Anandamurti, 'Subhasita Samgraha 13,' discourse: 'Subjective Approach and Objective Adjustment.')

4. Peterson, J. Quotation taken from the interview: 'Sir Roger Scruton/Dr. Jordan B. Peterson: Apprehending the Transcendent.'

5. 'According to general belief, psychology is a part of general science, and should therefore not be included as a part of philosophy. Thus psychology has been accepted as a

branch of science in the West... Yoga psychology, though a part of philosophy, is also a science, but is not restricted to the materialistic paradigm which characterizes Western philosophy and psychology. It is the science by which spiritual aspirants can acquire knowledge and mastery of themselves in their quest for Self-realization. Knowledge of yoga psychology is essential for spiritual practices; without this knowledge, aspirants will not achieve success in their spiritual endeavours.' (Anandamurti, 'Yoga Psychology,' chapter: 'Publisher's Note.)

6.   For example, in the song of the Baul, Sufi or other mystical-devotional traditions, in the songs of Tagore, or the compositions of Prabhat Samgiita by Anandamurti. (See: A.Tapasiddha, 2019)

7.   One of the earliest and most well-known examples is 'The Tao of Physics' by F. Capra. Other similar references include; the works of R. Sheldrake; 'The Eternal Dance of Macrocosm' by M. Towsey; or 'Microvita: Exploring a New Science of Reality', and 'From Imaginary Oxymora to Real Polarities and Return' by H.J. Rudolph, which attempts to explain the movement from consciousness to matter and idea to reality within the framework of mathematics.

8. 'This verse is in twilight language. On the surface there is one meaning and underneath another. The surface meaning is: "The courtyard went into the inner room – O honoured lady, do you understand? As a result of the courtyard going inside the room, the thief that was hiding in the courtyard also went inside and stole your earrings." The hidden meaning is: "By reaching the higher stages of spiritual practice the outer world is swallowed up within you. Then you also become all-knowing. That thief of minds has stolen away your worldly bondages."

On the practical level, what happens is that the unconscious mind is all-pervading, integral and immeasurably vast. Through spiritual practices the riches of the unconscious mind are brought down into the subconscious mind. The spiritual aspirant then understands everything; he discovers the secret signs of knowledge. Then, according to his or her needs, he or she is able to bring this acquired wealth of the subconscious mind into the conscious mind and use it in the external world.' (Anandamurti, 'Shabda Cayaniká Part 2', discourse: 'Indukamala to Iyatta.')

IISHVARA PRAN'IDHÁNA

1.   'There may be many interpretations of the term "Iishvara." But it commonly means "the controller of this universe". He who controls the thought-waves of this universe is Iishvara. Therefore, "Puruśottama" and "Iishvara" are not identical conceptions. In philosophy the word "Iishvara" has one more meaning – it is the witnessing counterpart of the objective Prakrti where the static principle is dominant. It is the witnessing entity of the causal world, it is the magnified essence of prájiṇa, it is an entity free from all bondages...

...Whatever may be the minor differences, to a sádhaka, Iishvara is understood to be nothing other than Saguńa Brahma or God.'   (Anandamurti, 'A Guide to Human Conduct.')

2.   'Pranidhana means to understand clearly or to adopt something as a shelter.' (Anandamurti, 'A Guide to Human Conduct.')

3. 'Hence Iishvara prańidhána means to let the entire psychic energy flow towards Iishvara as the object of Supreme ideation. (Anandamurti, 'Tattva Kaomudii Part 3.')

4. 'Saḿyoga yoga ityukto jiivátmá Paramátmanah – "When the unit consciousness merges itself fully and is finally identified with the Supreme Consciousness, Shiva, that is called yoga." (Anandmurti, 'Subhasita Samgraha Part 14,' discourse: 'Yoga, Tantra and Kevala Bhakti.')

5. Anandamurti, 'Subhasita Samgraha Part 1,' discourse: 'Yajina and Karmaphala.'

6.   This process is known as 'diiksa' or initiation: 'The imparting of proper spiritual training produces a spiritual awakening in the human mind, causing spiritual aspirants to seek that path which leads to the attainment of their iśta or spiritual goal. A competent spiritual teacher then will impart the practical guidance to those aspirants. That spiritual direction is called tántrikii diikśá. *'Tan jádyáta tárayeh yastu sah tantrah parikiirthita.'* The practical process which leads to the freedom from dullness is called Tantra. The process of initiation according to the science of tántra is called tantrik diikśá.' (Anandamurti, 'Tattva Kaomudii Part 2)

7. In Ananda Marga, an introductory meditation practice can be done using the kiirtan mantra (mantra used for spiritual chanting) until formal initiation is taken and a personal mantra is given. This introductory mantra is 'Baba Nam Kevalam' and means 'only the thought of infinite, divine consciousness' or 'everything is an expression of that divine consciousness.' It can be repeated mentally in rhythm with the respiration when seated cross-legged with the palms together in the lap and eyes closed. Further instruction can be taken from the acaryas of Ananda Marga.

8.   'The reported depth of meditation also corresponds to activity in the brain's pleasure centers, such as left forebrain bundle, anterior insula and precentral gyrus. This overt pleasure is accompanied by a shift in emotional self-regulation; meditators are more aware of thoughts and feelings conceptually, but less emotionally disrupted by them, according to one study. Both hemispheres are involved in self-observation.' (Webb, N. 'The Neurobiology of Bliss--Sacred and Profane.')

9. 'In the end, when its wavelength will, as well, become infinite, and those waves will also flow in a straight line, the mind will get transformed into the átman. This state is called samádhi. Here the psychic waves have attained a parallelism with the spiritual waves of the átman. This psycho-spiritual parallelism is known as "idea", or bháva. When this bháva or

idea is conceived on the psychic level, it is "ideology". Ideology, therefore, is the conception of idea and nothing else.

Hence when we call some materialistic or political principles of a person, party, nation or federation an "ideology", it is a wrong use of the term. "Ideology" involves in it a spiritual sense; it is an inspiration which has a parallelism with the Spiritual Entity.' (Anandamurti, 'Idea and Ideology,' chapter: 'Psycho-Spiritual Parallelism.')
10.

BIBLIOGRAPHY

-Aiyar, K.N. 1914. *'Thirty Minor Upanishads.'* Kessinger Publishing.

-Anandamurti, 2006. *'Ananda Marga: Elementary Philosophy.'* Electronic edition 7, Ananda Marga Pracaraka Samgha.

-Anandamurti. 2006. *'Ananda Sutram.'* Electronic edition 7, Ananda Marga Pracaraka Samgha.

-Anandamurti. 2006. *'Ananda Vacanamrtam Parts 3, 7, 14, 33.'* Electronic edition 7, Ananda Marga Pracaraka Samgha.

-Anandamurti. 2006. *'A Guide to Human Conduct.'* Electronic edition 7, Ananda Marga Pracaraka Samgha.

-Anandamurti. 2006. *'Caryacarya Parts 2 & 3.'* Electronic edition 7, Ananda Marga Pracaraka Samgha.

-Anandamurti. 2006. *'Discourses on Tantra Volume 2.'* Electronic edition 7, Ananda Marga Pracaraka Samgha.

-Anandamurti. 2006. *'Subhasita Samgraha Parts 1, 2, 7, 10, 13, 14, 18, 24.'* Electronic edition 7, Ananda Marga Pracaraka Samgha.

-Anandamurti. 2006. *'Tattva Kaomudii Part 2.'* Electronic edition 7, Ananda Marga Pracaraka Samgha.

-Anandamurti. 2006. *'Yoga Psychology.'* Electronic edition 7, Ananda Marga Pracaraka Samgha.

-Bharti. S.V. 2001. *'Yoga Sutras of Patanjali: With the Exposition of Vyasa.'* Delhi, Motilal Banarsidas.

-Bhattacharya, D. 1999. *'The Mirror of the Sky.'* Arizona, Hohm Press.

-Capra, F. 1981. *'The Tao of Physics.'* Suffolk, The Chaucer Press.

-Dostoyevsky, M. 1866. *'Crime and Punishment.'* Ebook, A-Z Classics.

-Dyczkowski, M. 1989. *'The Doctrine of Vibration.'* Delhi, Motilal Banarsidass.

-Huxley, A. 2002. *'Brave New World.'* Ebook, Project Gutenberg.

-'*Jordan Peterson vs Susan Blackmore: Do we need God to make sense of life?*' 2018. The Big Conversation from Unbelievable. (Youtube: https://www.youtube.com/watch?v=syP-OtdCIho)

-Lem, S. 1974. '*The Futurological Congress.*' Ebook. New York, The Continuum Publishing Corporation.

-Maturana, H. & Verden-Zoller, G. 2008. '*The origin of Humanness in the Biology of Love.*' Ebook. Exeter, Imprint Academic.

-Rudd, J. '*The Voice of Saruman: Wizards and Rhetoric in the Two Towers.*' (https://www.questia.com/library/journal/1G1-227196963/the-voice-of-saruman-wizards-and-rhetoric-in-the)

-Rudolf, H.J. 2011. '*From Imaginary Oxymora to Real Polarities and Return.*' Bloomington, Authorhouse.

-Rudolf, H. J. 2017. '*Microvita: Exploring a New Science of Reality.*' Bloomington, Authorhouse.

-'*Roger Scruton/Dr. Jordan B. Peterson: Apprehending the Transcendent.*' 2018, Cambridge. Presented by The Cambridge Centre for the Study of Platonism and Ralston College. (Youtube: https://www.youtube.com/watch?v=XvbtKAYdcZY)

-Rudreshvarananda. '*Uplifting Human Dignity in West Africa.*' (www.anandamarga.net/archive/rudreshvarananda.htm)

-'*Sacrifice.*' (https://en.wiktionary.org/wiki/sacrifice)

-Sarkar, P.R. 2006. '*A Few Problems Solved.*' Electronic edition 7, Ananda Marga Pracaraka Samgha.

-Sarkar, P. R. 2006. '*Idea and Ideology.*' Electronic edition 7, Ananda Marga Pracaraka Samgha.

-Sarkar, P. R. 2006. '*Neohumanism: The Liberation of Intellect.*' Electronic edition 7, Ananda Marga Pracaraka Samgha.

-Sarkar, P.R. 2006. '*Proutist Economics.*' Electronic edition 7, Ananda Marga Pracaraka Samgha.

-Sarkar, P.R. 2006. *'Shabda Cayanika Part 2.'* Electronic edition 7, Ananda Marga Pracaraka Samgha.
-Sepehri, S. 2013. *'A Selection of Poems from the Eight Books.'* Bloomington, Balboa Press.
-Shippey, T. 2010. *'JRR Tolkien: Author of the Century.'* London, Harper Collins.
-Singh, J. 2006. *'Vijnánabhairava or Divine Consciousness.'* Delhi, Motilal Banarsidass.
-Tagore, R. 1918. *'Nationalism.'* Ebook. London, Macmillan and Co.
-Tagore, R. 1916. *'Sadhana: The Realization of Life.'* Ebook, Project Gutenberg.
-Tolkien, J.R.R. 2000. *'The Letters of JRR Tolkien.'* London, Harper Collins.
-Tapasiddha, A. 2019. *'Ink of the Heart.'* Independently Published.
-Towsey, M. 2011. *'Eternal Dance of Macrocosm, Volume 2.'* Queensland, Proutist Universal.
-*'True Meaning of Brahmacarya.'* Art of Living. The Art of Living,' (https://www.artofliving.org/uy-es/yoga/patanjali-yogasutra/knowledge-sheet-70)
-Webb, N. 2011. *'The Neurobiology of Bliss--Sacred and Profane.'* Scientific American. (https://www.scientificamerican.com/article/the-neurobiology-of-bliss-sacred-and-profane/?redirect=1)
-Zamyatin, Y. 2013. *'We.'* Ebook. Sydney, Pan Macmillan.